Reclaiming Our Lives After Breast and Gynecologic Cancer

Kristine Falco, Psy.D.

JASON ARONSON INC.
Northvale, New Jersey
London

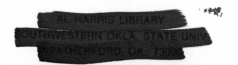

The author wishes to thank artist Kit Keith and medical consultant C. Diana Jordan, M.D. for the illustrations in Chapter 2.

Director of Editorial Production: Robert D. Hack

This book was set in 14 pt. Lapidary 333 by Alpha Graphics of Pittsfield, NH, and printed and bound by Book-mart Press, Inc. of North Bergen, NJ.

Library of Congress Cataloging-in-Publication Data

Falco, Kristine L.
    Reclaiming our lives after breast and gynecologic cancer /
Kristine Falco.
      p. cm.
    Includes bibliographical references and index.
    ISBN 0-7657-0099-9
    1. Cancer—Psychological aspects.   2. Women—Diseases—
Psychological aspects.   I. Title.
    RC281.W65F35   1997
    155.9'16'082—DC21   97-16795

Printed in the United States of America on acid-free paper. For information and catalog write to Jason Aronson Inc., 230 Livingston Street, Northvale, New Jersey 07647-1726. Or visit our website: http:/www.aronson.com

Reclaiming Our Lives After
Breast and Gynecologic Cancer

For all the brave women who've gone before
and the many still to come

Contents

Origins

The origins for my writing this book are twofold.

First, I am trained as a clinical psychologist who works with cancer patients.

Second, I am a woman who has had cancer. Breast cancer. Twice.

As a clinician, I have had the privilege—and hardship—of offering solace, information, skills, witnessing, and pathways of healing and renewal to all kinds of people with cancers and many other medical illnesses. I have received training to develop a specialization in an area of psychology that goes by several names: health psychology, behavioral health, and, the term I prefer, medical psychology. This special area of psychology concentrates on developing research and treatment methods that address the ways in which a person's medical condition is intertwined with his or her mental–emotional condition—and vice versa. Medical psychology works from the premise that our minds, our bodies, and our spirits are interactive and inseparable, each being influenced by the others.

I worked in the field of medical psychology long before my own cancer diagnosis. It has been very difficult, but very rewarding too, to provide the kind of aid that I do, helping people with acute distress over a recent, serious diagnosis, and helping people with more chronic, long term reevaluation and readjustment to medical conditions, including cancers, multiple sclerosis and other nervous system and muscular diseases, seizure disorders, diabetes, organ failure and transplants, paraplegia, athletic injuries, gastrointestinal disorders, lupus erythematosis, ALS (Lou Gerhig's Disease), fibromyalgia, and chronic fatigue syndrome.

I have had a lifelong interest in the intricate webbing that attaches our often-divided aspects—body, mind and thought, spirit, behavior, emotions—into a coherent and interactive whole. Occurrences in one of these areas affect the others, just as plucking one strand of a spider's web will move all the other strands to varying degrees as well. Which strands are moved, how much they are each moved, and whether each strand is strengthened or weakened or outright broken comprises the fabric of each individual person. This is the part I love the most about my work—discovering and working with the unique qualities of each strand of my patient's own web to guide the way to helping her the most.

My own cancer diagnosis came at age 38. I had just finished my doctoral studies and residency. I was living on

3 acres of country land my loved ones and I called "The Little Self-Sufficiency Farm," where I was chopping wood as the sole heat source, carrying water to the animals, growing many of my own vegetables and berries, tending a tiny fruit orchard, and caring for cats, horses, goats, ducks, chickens, geese, and turkeys, plus any wildlife that happened by, including the mother skunk who raised her young every year under my barn (and who sprayed me only once in 12 years when I came upon her suddenly and frightened her as she was teaching her kittens how to snitch food from the cats' dish).

At the time of my diagnosis, my first terror was of losing my life. The second was of losing my treasured independence—running that little farm. My femininity, too, felt in grave jeopardy. I beheld my ability to run that homestead much as the women pioneers had done—and as much earlier women ancestors who first began cultivating gardens had done. I was living in close cycles with the earth and her seasons, and doing so was an integral act of womanhood for me. Also, physically, I had smallish, perky breasts that I was very fond of (although, like most girls, I'd spent years thinking they were supposed to be bigger). I had to (or got to, depending on which hour you asked me) choose between mastectomy and lumpectomy, either of which, it seemed to me, would seriously deplete my sense of womanhood.

I spent marathon days talking to friends and loved ones, talking to breast cancer survivors, reading stacks of medical literature, writing my thoughts, and consulting with my farm animals (they can be a great channel of wisdom for me) and then chose a lumpectomy surgery. But the post-lumpectomy pathology study indicated that cancer cells were remaining right out to the edges of the removed lump tissue—a situation considered by most doctors at the time to be too risky to complete a cure by the radiation that often follows lumpectomy. So, one week later, I returned to the hospital for a mastectomy.

In just 3 weeks I'd gone from robust health through a biopsy and two major surgeries under depleting general anesthesia to end up one-breasted. Well! I was not pleased. But it didn't take me long to become pleased. And very determined. Determined especially to redefine and re-find my own femininity and womanhood, as well as personhood, as a big part of finding a new footing in life.

For me, a lot of my symbolism of femininity was associated with my breasts. From the incident at age 12 when I wadded tissues to help fill the cups of my first bra, I have watched and lovingly tended the growth and changes of what I saw as my most soft, bouncy, roundish, pliable, assertive sign of womanhood. By the way, the tissue in the bra was noticed, by my dad of all people, which embarrassed me enough to never do it again ("No false advertising," Dad said tenderly, Mom gently smiling nearby—a phrase I felt was rather sexist at the time). But now I think this came to help me feel just fine without reconstructive breast surgery and without prostheses. "No false advertising" became, in my mind, "It's great to be just who you are, to live well in your body just the way it is." Many difficult incidents indeed can be turned around to become very useful lessons and strengthening experiences.

Over the years, both before and after cancer, my vulva and pelvic organs also represented absolutely integral perceptions of myself as a womanly, feminine creature. My monthly menses feel to me to be signs of healthy operating systems. To lose these, as most pelvic cancer patients do, would call for yet another redefinition of my womanliness. And I *could* well lose them someday, to chemotherapy, to Tamoxifen, to metastatic breast cancer. Struggling with renewed perceptions of womanhood became a predominant part of my clambering to recovery, both physically and psychologically.

When I was just 2 months short of celebrating my 6-year cancer anniversary, my surgeon and I became concerned about a small lump in my remaining breast that seemed to have recently enlarged somewhat. Here we go again, I thought. Results of the needle aspiration biopsy were not conclusive, so a surgical biopsy was needed. This time, the biopsy procedure was familiar and for that reason only, it was a bit easier than the unforgettable biopsy of 6 years earlier. For the same reason, the several days' waiting time for this procedure was easier also. My surgeon said that the biopsy tissue she removed looked pretty healthy, so again I had a less difficult time waiting for the results of the pathology studies than I'd had before. Well, perhaps I'm exaggerating. Actually, these procedures and waiting times were emotionally exhausting and required my complete, loving attention, but they were indeed a bit less difficult than they had been before. Plus, I had statistics on my side. In my own case (and we're all unique in this way) my doctors and I had calculated about a 30% chance of ever having a cancer appear in my remaining breast. That's a 70% chance that I'll never have a cancer occurrence in the breast, for those of us who like to see the glass as half full.

But the pathologist found cancer. Again. The same kind as last time. I was thunderstruck. I was in the 30% group, not the 70% group as I'd hoped. Again, I set out to gather information, talk to people, and listen within myself so I could come up with the best choices for me. I was especially nonplussed to find that no real medical advances had occurred in the 6 years since my first cancer. Medical science had learned virtually nothing new in those 6 years to improve treatment, to improve diagnostics, to improve knowledge of who belonged in which treatment groups.

So, I faced the same decisions again. Should I have a mastectomy? Or a lumpectomy with radiation? Or the more risky lumpectomy without radiation? Should I have a lymph node dissection this time too? Will I forgo chemotherapy this time again? And forgo Tamoxifen treatment? I read, I cried, I talked, I felt alternately overwhelmed and very strong, I turned to my spiritual guides, and I even got a second opinion pathology report. (Your doctor can send your biopsy tissue to a second pathologist if you ask—and because cancer is not always easily diagnosable, I recommend doing so whether your diagnosis is a cancer or not.) I felt quite strongly that I wanted to keep the one breast I still had—it was to me such an important piece of my femininity. Yet, the clear voice from deep inside kept reminding me that I apparently have breast tissue that is prone to growing cancers—and the recommended post-lumpectomy radiation is not foolproof.

With a heavy heart, but a feeling that this was right for me, I chose mastectomy. Breastless at age 44. How can this happen? But it did. Again I chose no chemotherapy. In Stage I breast cancer, chemotherapy only saves about 3 lives out of 100. Another gamble I'd make. And I chose no Tamoxifen, since the research says it helps more if you're postmenopausal, which I wasn't, and it helps prevent recurrences of cancer in the breasts themselves, which I no longer would have, more than it helps prevent recurrence in other organs. And I did choose to have a sampling lymph node dissection done because I would change my mind about having chemotherapy if there were any cancer cells in the lymph nodes. There weren't!

I had thought all this would be so much easier if it were to ever happen a second time, having done it all before. It was indeed easier in some ways: The medical information was clear to me and what I was likely to feel and need was more comprehensible to me, so I could plan well for all the nurturing and all the information I would need. The physical recovery took longer, I've guessed, because I was just enough older the second time to notice a difference in my body's ability to quickly replenish itself. But the actual experience of cancer again was no easier at all. There is just no way I can make this okay, I felt.

So I held on for the ride and kept cultivating a trust in myself that I would carry through finding a way to integrate this, that I would find a way to embrace my experiences with cancer yet emerge with inward wholeness and zestfulness. Indeed, I am accomplishing this. A big surprise to me—one I never would have predicted—is that I really, really like what I see in the mirror each day. I see a slender, fit, boyish, breastless (and nipple-less) strong body that can still do anything I'm willing to train it to do. I can ride horses and hike and ride bikes and garden and teach and write and provide psychological services and sing and laugh and run and ski and practice yoga and make love and lounge around and chop wood and learn new things and cook great meals and play musical instruments and care for my loved ones and my animals just as much as I like. This is enough for me. In fact, this feels like a very rich life indeed.

Yes, I miss my breasts. And I wish this had all never happened. And I live with the heavy thought that if there's a next time for me, the cancer will by definition be in a more lethal location than in both times past. But I really do like my body and its capabilities. And I feel that I now embody a new kind of femininity. This femininity includes that boyish-looking chest (and it's always good to incorporate some desirable masculine traits in our feminine self-concept) that I had for the first 10 years or so of my life. It's a chest that makes me think of the childhood freedoms of climbing trees and hanging from my knees on the bars in the school yard—good feelings. At the same time, this renewed femininity incorporates an image of myself as the epitome of the graceful older woman that I hope to become, a concept of myself as a sprightly and rooted more elderly woman whose breasts would have begun to change from plump to lean by this time anyway, just like they're supposed to. And

I never need reminding that each day, each experience, and each person can be sumptuous to me. This path and this view are working well for me, and it is part of what inspires my clinical practice.

In my psychology practice, I have worked with many patients who have had breast or gynecologic cancers and many patients (male and female) whose mothers, aunts, siblings, wives, and even grown children have had women's cancers or have had the scare of a breast lump or a pelvic mass. Rarely do these people speak of threats to femininity in a direct way. Rather, these aspects of cancer's effects arise from the deep waters of concern about related topics such as sexuality, touchability, desirability, attractiveness, fears of freakishness or of being badly scarred, reluctance about nudity, lack of purpose, loss of identity, and loss of role. As these concerns are looked at from the breadth of view they deserve in psychotherapy, it is apparent to me that each concern comprises spokes of a wheel and that the hub of that wheel is the cancer survivor's shaken sense of womanhood. But it is a womanhood that indeed can be reclaimed.

Helping women make a reclamation of their womanhood is the goal of much of the psychotherapeutic work I do. Thus, this book. Women, and their therapists, need more expression and synthesis of this aspect of having a woman's cancer—the cancer's effects on one's sense of femininity and womanhood. It is clear to me that both breast cancer and pelvic cancers have a tendency to create a seismic shake-up in the landscape of a woman's sense of herself as feminine. Further, it is clear to me that each woman may experience her femininity in ways that are unique to her. It is in the discovery, letting go, and remaking of these ways that survivors of women's cancers remake their lives, usually for the better.

If you have had a woman's cancer or worry that you will ever have one, if someone you love has had a woman's cancer, or if you are a professional who works with women with these cancers, this book is for you. In these pages we will look at the effects—short term and long term—that having a woman's cancer has on a woman, her sense of self, her femininity, her liveliness, her coping abilities, her relational aptitudes, and her need to rethink her own values and rules about womanhood.

For women with cancer, or those who love them, my hope is that this book will provide you with substantive information to help you on your cancer pathways as well as substantive concepts for the deep work that can be required in order to reemerge from cancer with an eventual renewed vision of your womanhood. If you are a woman with a woman's cancer, this book may be a beam of light to illuminate the really incredible number of feelings, effects, expectations, and experiences you may encounter along your cancer travels. It is intended to help you understand the choices you will have of treatments and of lifestyle and of how to make your own light of your womanhood shine renewed.

If you are close to a woman who has a woman's cancer, this book will show you many viewpoints and provide a plentitude of information to help you be a companion and witness to your loved one's cancer experience.

If you are a professional who works with women who have women's cancers—a psychologist, physician or psychiatrist, social worker, counselor, nurse, body worker, spiritual worker, or member of a similar profession—this book will provide you with templates for guiding your work with these women patients. I hope this book serves as a foundation for understanding many of the psychological dynamics that are likely to be manifest in your patients and clients, which will in turn help with assessment and treatment planning. The writing is addressed to a woman who has cancer herself, but I have described the issues in ways that give a therapist or other professional clear road maps of necessary information, experiential issues, and directions for healing to inform the therapeutic process.

I offer heartfelt thanks to the many people whose love and encouragement have lit my path. The alchemy of the energy that these people shine on me is a wonder, transforming as it does into the needed forms of inspiration and vitality. I thank you, my family, friends far and near, loved ones who are still in this life and those who are not, and the many wonderful and brave cancer patients who have shared their struggles, hopes, and reclamations with me.

1

Womanhood
and Cancer

All cancers are devastating. A diagnosis of cancer is consuming, frightening, and exhausting to its new owner. Abundant numbers of good books, organizations, and support systems are now available to promote a well-informed voyage through the initial, shocking forecast of cancer and through its often lengthy aftermath. While there are indeed many books on coping with cancer, this book is different. It is about specific cancers afflicting women, cancers that afflict us in those areas of our bodies that have important, personalized, psychological meanings. This is a book about cancers of the breast and gynecologic organs—that is, cancers of the uterus, ovaries and fallopian tubes, cervix, vagina, and vulva. These are women's cancers.

Breast cancers and gynecologic (or pelvic) cancers affect more than just a woman's physiology, more than her body.

These cancers can affect her very sense of herself. They can have a deep impact on her image of herself and of her purpose and place in life. These women's cancers especially can make an indelible, new imprint on a woman's view of her own femininity, of her womanhood.

The "Rules of Womanhood," so to speak, in all cultures are conveyed to a female beginning in young girlhood and continuing throughout her lifetime. Some of these rules may never have been spoken outwardly, yet they become subliminally ingrained as subconscious daily expectation, behavior, and context to a woman's life. A woman who has a woman's cancer is no exception to the effects of these rules: some good effects, some not so good. Many women would say that the major rules of womanhood might be: Be Attractive, Be a Lady, Be Unselfish, Make Relationships Work Well, Put Others First, and Be Competent Without Complaint. I am sure that none of these "rules" are any surprise to women readers. But most importantly, these rules can be shaped, and reshaped, by each woman in ways that can reduce their inherent constrictions and expand their application instead to areas of her life and her own traits that she values.

> *Having a woman's cancer gives one many opportunities to rethink these rules.*

WOMANHOOD: SELF, BODY, CULTURE, AND IDENTITY

What is womanhood? I recently asked a group of women to write down for me their symbolic, associative meanings to womanhood and femininity. Here is what this group of women had to say:

Womanhood to these woman conjured ideas of *strength, aliveness, vulnerability, fecundity, fertility, power, creativity, softness, endurance, resilience, resourcefulness, sisterhood, and nurturing.* When I tallied the number of times that each of these words was used (the women had written their responses on cards to hand in), one word appeared far more often than any of the others. That word was "strength." To these women, womanhood means mostly strength.

The word *Femininity* made these women think of terms such as *submission, attractiveness, relational abilities, grace, weakness, beauty, frivolous, nurturing, helplessness, softness, artificiality, not taking a stand, living only for others, gentleness, generosity, warmth, dresses, delicate, self-conscious, a "nice girl," passive, and pretty.* The most common term associated with femininity was "weak."

I was struck by the dichotomy here. Many people would see the terms "femininity" and "womanhood" as similar in meaning. Yet, at least to this group, the two terms do have a few overlapping characteristics, such as nurturing and softness, but have quite opposite meanings at their core: Womanhood means strength, femininity means weakness.

I think this expresses a profound truth. Women are encouraged to be both weak and strong. Indeed, we humans are all both strong and weak. Occurring at the same time, or during different waves of our lives, we are strong and we are weak. I think it is only when we have not yet had a chance to think about our strong areas and our areas of weakness, our strong times and our weak times, that this becomes a problem. Women who encounter a women's cancer are given the chance to really explore—and redecide—how and where it is good to be strong and how and where it is okay, and real, to be weak.

For example, some of women's strengths have been traditionally undervalued or trivialized, while some of our weaknesses have been extolled. This is a very confusing state of affairs; women are being handed a map to follow that is contradictory and therefore seemingly impossible. This is not how things have to be. And the experience of cancer can open our eyes to a new way to notice these constricting and backwards ways, to reevaluate them for ourselves, to embrace both our strength and our weakness, and to renew our own definitions of womanhood and femininity.

Think about the example of "feminine intuition." This way of "knowing" some things about the world is too often thought of as silly or irrational. Instead, we might come to think of feminine intuition as an ability to embrace our dependent qualities more easily, thereby developing an ability to relate in nonrational, nonlogical modes, such as with gestures and the use of implied and emotional expressions—and to infer personal meaning from a wide range of signals often otherwise ignored. What has been pejoratively labeled "feminine intuition" can instead be seen as a sixth sense, an ability to read information from people and situations that is neither spoken directly nor deduced by logic only.

Think also about a woman's emotional expressiveness. Our emotional expressiveness is often dismissed as an irrational result of hormonal fluctuations or as a method we use to intentionally manipulate others. Instead, we may come to view our emotional expressiveness as a vital and poetic narration of feelings, as an indicator of advanced psychological development. Open expressions of differentiated and modulated feelings serve women in understanding that, contrary to popular Western belief, emotional dependence is basic to human life.

Thirdly, think also about the assumption that female development typically includes a concern for personal beauty, an aesthetic orientation to everyday life, which may be trivialized by commercial pandering of cosmetics manufacturers. Alternatively, when a woman has consciously integrated the power of her appearance as an aspect of her authentic identity, she comes into control of a wide range of choices about how to express herself (Young-Eisendrath and Weidemann 1987).

Other common sex-role stereotypes suggest that women should be dependent, portraying us as lost and helpless without a male partner and seeing us as more attractive if we enhance "little girl" qualities. We encounter intense pressure to look eternally adolescent rather than motherly, or matronly, or womanly. Even personality traits of infancy and childhood are encouraged (while simultaneously disdained) in women; crying, whining, seductiveness, manipulation, and petulance are viewed as common and acceptable ways for women to make their demands met. Women, like children, are seen to have considerable emotionality. Sexual naiveté and innocence are encouraged, and being sexually experienced is not. Adult females are pressured to remain *girls* (that is, to cultivate adorable, innocent, childlike, dependent features) and behave like *ladies* (that is, to adhere to values of gentility, propriety, cleanliness, impulse control, and conformity to social norms). Even the word *woman* seems to infer too much strength or power or dominance or worth to be seemly; the word is used only infrequently in every day speech. *Girls, gals,* or *ladies* are terms used much more often, and they do not connote as much strength as the word *woman*.

Most sadly, intellectual mastery and skill are progressively discouraged. "Be smart enough to catch a man, but never outsmart him" is a message sent often covertly and sometimes overtly to women. We are taught to make ourselves pretty or attractive enough to be *sought after* rather than to actively pursue what we want. Television, books, and magazines too often portray women as silly, gossipy, capricious, illogical, and intellectually helpless. The Western norm is that heterosexual men don't seek female partners who are their intellectual equal or superior. Indeed, think about how many *male nurse–female doctor* couples you know of compared to the other way around. How many *female lawyer–male legal assistant* couples? How many *female foreman–male line worker* couples? How many of any such mixtures are seen in the popular media?

Girls and women are still subtly discouraged from entering traditionally male occupations and academic fields, and those women who manage to get there often report finding the work atmosphere so unpleasant as to make leaving the field a viable, even personally healthy, consideration. Another still-common stereotype is that physical strength and prowess are considered unattractive in women. We are taught to exaggerate, even pretend, weakness and delicacy and to enlist men to take care of us. Also, men rarely seek women partners who are stronger or taller than they. Nor do women seek men who are less strong or shorter than they.

These and other aspects of womanhood can come into question as we encounter the impact of a woman's cancer. And, hopefully, the outcome can be a redefinition and enhancement of who each of us is—as an individual woman and in relation to others who inhabit our world. The definitions of womanhood and femininity that were transmitted to each of us can become narrowing and rigid if they are left unexamined, but they can become a broadened, enriched reclamation of traits that are of value, and traits that make room for the entire gamut of human abilities, including those traits that are traditionally considered masculine.

In this self-examination and self-evaluation process, each woman can decide for herself where she can be strong and where she may be weak; further, she can make well-thought decisions about how to best use her strengths and about what kind of aid to seek for needed bolstering in her weaker areas. Notice that the goal here is not to become completely strong in every area; rather, a woman's goal is to cultivate and use strengths according to her values and to invent plans and supportive networks to provide reinforcements in her areas of lesser skill, lesser strength, lesser stamina. Each of us will always have both our strengths and our weak places. A woman lives well who can know these parts of herself and work within them, lovingly and wisely, rather than expecting herself to become A+ competent in every possible sector. Asking for help and building a network of resources for the weaker areas is just as important—and healthy—as knowing and using the areas of strength.

Having a woman's cancer can slap us right in the face with a startling awareness of these principles. After the diagnosis, we are never the same again. In the fallout, the very definition of our femininity is drawn into question as we struggle with learning new ways to be strong, new ways to ask for help, new ways to develop our sense of femininity, of womanhood.

Not a small number of my women cancer patients tell me they each have no clue how to receive help from others. Each realizes that she operates on the—heretofore unchallenged—belief that she can only allow herself to be helped if it seems medically or physically necessary—such as being driven home after a treatment that makes her too ill to drive by herself, or only being able to turn down an unwanted invitation or request because she can say she doesn't feel well enough to do it. But so often she has to really work at her definitions of womanhood, dependence, selfishness, and related topics before she can make new decisions about what it means to receive others' help when it isn't physically necessary. The goal is to gratefully and gracefully be able to receive such kind "unnecessary" help as being bathed, being driven to appointments even when you can do it yourself, having a companion in the waiting room just because it feels nice, letting someone else do some research for you or fetch you something, or, perhaps the hardest kind, turning down a request or an invitation just because you'd rather not do it this time.

THE BODY

In the world of women in Western culture, a great deal of emphasis is placed on a woman's body. Only firm and unlined bodies are deemed attractive. The shape, texture, look, and attractiveness of the body is paraded at great length in most arenas that we are exposed to: television, magazines, movies, radio programs, advertisements, popular music, and the like. Cancer, too, is often regarded primarily as a bodily experience.

Of course, a woman comprises a lot more than just her body. And women's cancers perhaps prove that point—poignantly and pointedly. While we may choose to make our bodies attractive, cancer often helps us redefine that attractiveness. A new definition may include not only outward attractiveness to the standards of other people we choose to appreciate us, but to our own standards as well—possibly changing our meaning of attractiveness to include an athletic look, a particular agility, a strength of purpose, a shine in our eyes that reflects inner peace, facile hands that play a musical instrument or create art or dote on children, a posture of body that invites closeness to others, and so on.

A woman is too often judged and given worth by her appearance, not by her strength, health, or ability to act effectively, not by her body's speed or endurance or ability but its shape and size. If her appearance is deemed desirable, then so is she, and she is treated accordingly. If her body is not deemed desirable, then she is worth less—even worthless. She may then be ridiculed or attacked; after all, by her very appearance she is considered to be asking for it:

It is assumed that she has chosen to be unattractive and deserves to be treated badly for it. She *is* her appearance. Heavy women tell very common horror stories of being ridiculed by strangers, told what to (not) eat in restaurants, and called names while walking along the street.

The *hypervisibility* for women of physical appearance and desirability results, paradoxically, in a heightened sense of *invisibility*. If the apparatus through which one experiences one's life is consistently being evaluated and is judged not by how well it works but by how well it pleases the perceiver, then the most important question is not "How well does my body work?" but "How do I appear to you?" The answer to "How are you?" becomes "I don't know. You tell me" (Kashack 1992). These constrictive definitions can be examined and changed. A woman's cancer can be the catalyst.

If women are deemed "fashion crazy" it is not because we are frivolous but perhaps because we have been led to believe that our bodies are our only power. We therefore take our bodies as seriously as men are encouraged to take their jobs. If a woman's body is her only real asset, it is thus also her greatest liability, a guarantee of inevitable defeat. The female body grows old, ceases to reproduce, loses its beauty (as it is culturally defined), and fades in its power. If a woman's power is centered in her body, so ultimately will be her powerlessness.

Her body is not seen as belonging to her but is appropriated by and for others (Rosser 1994). It is in danger of becoming an object for the use of others, especially men, whether in providing heirs or sexual service or adornment or physical labor in return for needed bodily protection.

And this needed bodily protection is really a result of the vicious circle of having kept her body in a soft and vulnerable state in order to attract a man, which therefore renders a woman too soft and vulnerable to protect herself if she were to need to.

A teenage immigrant to the United States describes it this way:

> My shoulders stoop, I nod frantically to indicate my agreement with others, I smile sweetly at people to show I mean well, and my chest recedes inward so that I don't take up too much space, so that I am not noticed—mannerisms of a marginal, off-centered person who wants both to be taken in and to fend off the threatening others. [Hoffman 1989]

Women are often characterized, both in popular and in psychological contexts, as being preoccupied with their appearance. Preoccupation with personal beauty has been analyzed in all sorts of areas to mean such things as compensation for a missing penis, fear of achievement, inferior thinking, inferior physical strength, or lack of material resources. "Women's narcissism," as it is often called, is commonly thought to be a substitution for something more genuinely worthwhile. But these theories of feminine narcissism are nonsense; they fail to account for the social context in which a woman's appearance is the only socially condoned form of power openly afforded her (Young-Eisendrath and Weidemann 1987).

In some of the worst manifestations of stereotyped womanhood, women are given the contradiction to be seen and not be seen. To be seen by men is considered the highest compliment, one which we should *elicit*, yet not *solicit*. That is, we must try to obtain something by not looking like we are actually reaching for it. We are not to be seen, in the manner of being too loud, nor demanding that our needs be honored, nor being too flamboyant, nor standing up for ourselves.

After a diagnosis of a woman's cancer, these under-the-surface issues can create a strong undertow current; the cancer, its surgical changes, its emotional aftermath, its effect on self-image and identity all are under contradictory dictums to both be shown ("Just cry and let it all out, dear") and not shown ("She's taking this all so well, going on as if nothing has happened"). This is a tough course to navigate, one that can only be done well when a woman has taken the time to examine for herself the effects and the meaning of these opposing codes in her own life.

If women sometimes feel contradictory or empty, it is reflective of the characteristic feminine project of trying to achieve self-affirmation through self-negation. For example, a woman's course is to feel worthy by denying herself, feel feminine by effacing herself, or, for some, to become a compulsive eater, trying to get herself simultaneously more and less visible (Greenspan 1983).

> I don't like to put on makeup, and these elaborate preparations are disturbing to me, as if we were in a harem and remodeling ourselves into a

special species—girls—so that we can appeal to that other, alien species, boys. They are supposed to come and get us, of course, but only after we have made ourselves into these appetizing and slightly garish bonbons. In the conspiratorial giggles in the room, there is the murmur of an unspoken agreement: we're not going to show them who we are, we're going to show them what they want. [Hoffman 1989]

In much of the Arab world, an ideal woman's body is a rounded body with broad hips and a gently curved stomach sloping down to the thighs, uninterrupted by any bony protrusions. A woman's body is seen as being suited mostly for bearing children, providing nourishment, and keeping children warm in the folds of flesh. It is also for feeding and satisfying a man's lust. Many other cultures have stereotyped images of an ideal woman that at least avoids the unhealthy focus on thinness that is so prominent in the West, but these definitions often yield yet another narrow definition of what a woman's body is supposed to look like. The resulting aspirations leave countless women in a context where their bodies may not naturally match.

If we add to this situation the internal and external bodily changes of cancer treatments, we are left with a potentially disastrous circumstance. The crisis of having a woman's cancer may bend the branches of a woman's sense of self completely to the ground, as she may feel less and less that she meets the former definition of femininity because of surgeries, radiation, chemotherapy, scars, pain, poor health, and drugs. These bent branches, however, may raise back up to the sky, even spring higher than ever before, as she grapples with new notions of womanhood and of who she is to herself and to those around her.

Cancer is a paradigm affecting the relationship of a woman to her body, regardless of whether there is an actual diagnosis or not. Breasts, for example, may have become a "lost innocence" (Oxenhandler 1995). In these times of alarmingly high breast cancer risk, breasts are often experienced as an ongoing source of uncertainty, a potential site of malignant growth, rather than as valued body parts to be appreciated for their function or their sexual responsiveness or their signal of womanliness. All girls and women are now faced with the task of generating a language, an imagery, a voice that might help us live with the simultaneous preciousness and vulnerability of our breasts. Women usually experience breast cancer with savagery and betrayal. And we experience the dread of it with a sad mistrust of our breasts.

What we must navigate is an authentic and empowering way to live with the breasts' inherent contradictions— as that which is simultaneously cherished, threatened, and threatening, the site of pleasure that can so readily give rise to the seed of danger. Unlike in previous generations, little girls whose adult family members have had breast and pelvic cancers may know of their own risk for cancer from early on in their lives. What impact this must have for these girls on their sense of femininity and womanhood as they mature and especially as they develop menarche and breasts!

The breasts do have a clear function: they are designed for feeding the young. This basic anatomic-physiologic definition has been eclipsed by the emotional and cultural values placed on the breasts, which minimize their basic function, that is, the production of milk. For several decades in the middle of this century, most Western children were not fed a single drop of breast milk. As a result of Western cultural expectations, breasts have become more symbolic than functional, coming to represent femininity and sexuality. It is often reported that the sight of a woman's breast has greater sexual arousal than a view of her genitalia (Small 1994).

The female breast is so idealized that it is often the primary focus of a woman's identification with the feminine role. For the young girl, an early awareness has emphasized that the appearance of her breasts is a measure of her desirability and acceptability as a woman. She subliminally interprets her own development in terms of the cultural expectations, so that no matter what her actual breast configuration, the tendency is for her to be dissatisfied if her breasts do not meet the current standards.

This type of body image dissatisfaction has led to the evolution of a large industry that provides prosthetic breast augmentation and reconstruction. This speaks to the driving motive to meet a body image standard without serious consideration of risk, psychological and physical (Small 1994). So strong is the cultural emphasis on breast form that many relatives of breast cancer survivors have had breast enhancement surgery despite the fact that they are at high risk for cancer due to the family history and despite the fact that these implants will make it harder for them to detect a lump should a cancer ever occur. We live in a society that worships breasts, not for their function, but for their form

(Runcowicz and Haupt 1995). That is not to say that I think function is more important than form. Rather, both function and form can be valuable, coexisting perspectives.

In past generations, children were not usually taught the biology and anatomy of sexuality, and they were left to such discoveries on their own; males had, and still do have, an advantage here of being allowed to handle their sexual organs on a regular basis for urination. Even in the current somewhat more liberated times, girls are still only told part of the story. Girls are told "boys have penises, girls have vaginas," (or worse, girls have just wombs). This is a failure to explicitly acknowledge and label our external genitalia, our vulvar area—the labia, the urinary opening, and especially the clitoris. This can impair a girl's capacity to develop an accurate psychic representation or map of her genitals and impede her ability to make differentiated judgments about both pleasurable sexual activities and potential disease processes (Lerner 1988). An encounter with a gynecologic cancer will almost certainly drive home a new or renewed awareness of both internal and external anatomic and functional genitalia.

For a woman who has never had the opportunity to "correct" an inaccurate psychic map of her genitalia and reproductive organs, a gynecologic cancer and its treatments can prove particularly puzzling or agreeably illuminating. To lose these body parts just as they are being discovered can be a most unhappy experience. Of course, losing them even when one has had a full appreciation of them for many years is also likely to bring unhappiness, at least for a time. Some changes in sexual pleasure are inevitable but not always in-surmountable. Changes for a woman in a more internalized sense of herself as a sexual being are also inevitable, but again the crisis of the cancer can open an opportunity for a re-evaluation of each woman's evolving values. Becoming unable to have children may be only one of several important aspects of the changes that can come from treatment for gyneco-logic cancers or chemotherapy treatment for breast cancer. Internalized sense of fertility, purpose, womanliness, and attractiveness as well as her experience of herself as sexually desirable and of having sexual desire of her own—all these are up for reevaluation upon dealing with a woman's cancer.

This whole issue of women's bodies and attractiveness is full of contradictory values and confounding priorities. To wit, many articles appear in the literature for women with cancer on subjects such as "How To Look Good During Cancer Treatment." I have mixed feelings about this sort of approach. On one hand, I think it is great for women to have information on how to incorporate wigs, hats, scarves, head wraps, jewelry and other accessories, products for dry treated skin, breast prostheses, and special makeup in order to feel less freakish during chemotherapy or radiation treatment. It can be a good thing to work toward feeling good about one's self and changing the (potentially negative) impact of others' reactions to us when we look unwell. On the other hand, these treatments *do* make us very sick, and it goes against my "honesty grain" to present cancer and its treat-ments as merely a problem of dress and cosmetics. The bad side of this approach can promote a woman's own negation of the deep meaning of what she is going through, thus preventing her from the very reevaluation of her values that can be cancer's greatest gift.

Attempting to look as if nothing important is happening to her can also promote lack of self awareness and prevent others from offering love or aid for the woman with cancer. And in the broader picture, it contributes to the sense of aloneness and freakishness that each newly diagnosed woman experiences, precisely because she has seen so very few models of women bravely reconstituting their lives—looking as ill as they really are while doing so. Perhaps there are times to be looking one's best and adorning oneself with accessories that make us feel "normal" or attractive and other times to be fully authentic and congruent with any illness we are experiencing and with our fears showing in our sallow but brave faces.

For many, many of the patients I have worked with, the act of removing a head wrap is a profoundly important deed. For her, just to be there, with her therapist, hairless head bared, soul shining through her eyes, scared and courageous, becomes a life-affirming feat. These acts say so much, especially to the patient herself. She almost always starts smiling, very broadly. I am there with her, a witness, not scared away by what I see; as a matter of fact, I am drawn deeply to this new sight. Her countenance speaks loudly, sometimes for the first time in her whole life, that it is her spirit, her self that can be beautiful, that she can glow from within with the radiance of life that still courses through her, regardless of any concept of a number of days or years remaining to her.

When she puts her wrap or wig back on her head, it is with new perspective. No longer is it to hide, an expression of embarrassment, an inconsolable sorrow. The head covering now becomes more freely chosen, a temporary adornment that she can use when she wants to and not when she doesn't want to. She has taken possession of her bald state; it no longer has possession of her.

TO CHERISH SELF AND OTHERS

Traditional notions of love imply that a woman should set herself aside, that she should sacrifice herself unconditionally rather than in the more healthy manner of choosing appropriate sacrifice that fits the situation. In the traditional mode, caring is seen not as love and generativity and power and passion but as passive and "giving with the self left out" (Bepko and Krestan 1993). There are two kinds of vulnerability that women raised in our society tend to have. The first is the quality of self-sacrifice, a learned willingness to set our own interests aside and to be used, and even used up, by the community. The second is a readiness to believe messages of disdain and derogation rather than seeing ourselves as worth defending, using the anger that arises at the disdain and derogation as a signal to take care, stand up, or move away from the source of disregard (Bateson 1989).

Concepts of what it means to be a woman are often concocted from notions of frivolous, empty-headed pleasure seekers pursuing sexual goals, plus an image of the dependent drudge condemned to sweeping floors or to a boring

24-hour-a-day care of children. Half consciously it all adds up to a choice between being concubine and slave. The first she despises, the second she fears, or vice versa, and thus she can be miserably caught in an interpretation of womanhood as a choice between using men or being used by them. "Yet the instinct of the feminine is precisely to *use* nothing, but simply to give and receive" (Luke 1995). Having a woman's cancer may help turn these notions on their heads and allow re-creation of definitions of love and giving that include being as loving toward ourselves as we are toward the others who are meaningful to us.

It is not easy to learn to cherish oneself when one's life has been organized around cherishing others, or when all the cherishing has been delegated to someone else. Self-care is important for health and stress reduction, but it is important for its own sake as well. It is intimately tied to self-esteem, with the implication that the one who is cherished is important and valuable—a message that our inward selves really takes seriously. "Care-taking is part of the composition of almost every life" (Bateson 1989). In this society, we habitually underestimate the impulse in men, women, and even children to care for one another and their need to be taken care of.

The best caretaker is one who offers a combination of challenge and support. To be nurturing is not always to concur and comfort, to stroke and flatter and appease; often, it requires offering a caring version of the truth, grounded in reality. Self-care should include the cold shower as well as the scented tub. Real caring requires setting priorities and limits (Bateson 1989), both for ourselves and for those we care about.

Women are not only encouraged to please others, to not hurt others, but many of us really *like* living by these values—"hurt no one, if you can help it." This can be a great philosophy of life, but it gets us into trouble if we forget to include *ourselves* in the list of people whom we shouldn't be hurtful to. Being too much of a pleaser can be a problem, in life and in cancer. For one thing, it can lead to a reluctance to ask questions, to ask for more information, to ask why. And it can cause a reluctance to resolve complaints, for fear of being (a) disliked, (b) seen as selfish for putting ourselves first, or (c) treated with retaliation or indifference or less than optimally. We may be especially fearful of irritating the doctor, thinking she or he will quit giving us the best possible treatment in return.

Women are often described as too involved in their relationships to others, in what others think, in what others want. This is another one of those traits that isn't all bad, and really should be cultivated, but should also be counterbalanced with enough independence and self-sufficiency to feel whole and secure. Western societies tout the fallacy of independence and rugged individualism. But many women organize their identity—and find meaning—within actual or internalized relational contexts rather than by being the rugged individualist (Jordan and Surrey 1986). It is not women's need for affiliation or her relationship orientation that predisposes women to a state of depletion or depression, as is often suggested in psychological literature—

because emotional connectedness is a basic human need as well as a strength. Rather, it is what *happens* to women in relationships that deserves our attention (Lerner 1988). A cancer will often bring these issues into a very front-and-center status.

Women do tend to meet others' needs before nurturing themselves. Also, we may expect that just as we see another's need and try to fill it, they will do the same for us. Quite the opposite usually happens, because a relationship has a tendency to go further and further into its original design, with a giver being expected to keep giving, and give more. Then, when we realize that our own needs aren't being well met, we are prone to starting to believe that our needs must not really be very important. So we end up either believing we don't need or deserve being nurtured or that self-nurturing should be last on our list of things to do (Louden 1992).

Why nurture ourselves? Because self-nurturing is vital. Women take care of others every day—sometimes when we should not but haven't yet examined the cost of this type of over-giving, sometimes because we want to, and sometimes because we place value on what we give and to whom. It is a very good idea to turn our wonderful nurturing ability toward ourselves as well as toward others.

Self-nurturing is an essential ingredient for healthy, authentic relationships, not a selfishness. It is essential to nurture ourselves and to obtain nurturing from many outside sources, if we honestly want to nurture the people we care about. It's a myth that we are endless vessels of giving. What about the need to go get filled back up so we have more to give? We cannot nurture others from a dry well. We need to take care of our own needs, too. And sometimes first! Then we can give from our surplus so much more deeply and abundantly to others. Our giving will then feel richly and freely given, without strains of resentment or exhaustion or hurry. During a cancer experience is an optimal time to become especially good at taking in nurture, from ourselves and from others. It can be a time to be cared for and to replenish depleted reserves, both so that we can return to the most vibrant health possible and so that we can give to others again from a place of "plenteousness."

VITALITY

Akin to the concept of unselfish self-nurturing is the notion of seeing to it that we are obtaining frequent refreshment and replenishment. Everything we do is necessarily limited by finite resources of simply being a human creature; yet the capacity to mobilize those physical resources depends on "psychic energy," or vitality. The physical energy to act may come from good rest and nutrition, but the "inner energy" or psychic energy can come from a flower or a sunset or laughter or a remembered smile.

An activity that increases vitality does not directly subtract from energy to do other activities—often it will enhance them instead. Take the example of exercise: On the one hand, physical effort can be depleting, even exhausting; on the other hand, regular exercise leads to the feeling of having more energy available, a more efficient metabolism, and a more alert mind. This notion holds true in many areas of life; maintaining vitality is an important element for being able to be creative and productive (Bateson 1989).

Thus, just as it is good for us to seek nurturing, it is good for us to seek the replenishing activities that bring vitality. This is so during cancer treatments, and, of course, for the rest of our lives. For some women, this is a new challenge, to actively seek that which brings us the things we value.

One patient of mine exemplifies dedication to creating refreshment and replenishment in her life. She is a breast cancer survivor with two high-school-age children who tends to the children and home while her husband earns the family income, an arrangement she likes very much now that she has reevaluated her life post-cancer. Prior to her cancer, she described her life as a stay-at-home-mom as unstimulating and exhausting. What has changed is her post-cancer project of developing a multitude of refreshing and replenishing activities. As she describes it, "I treat myself as if I were one of the most important, precious people I know." She is careful to get the rest and sleep she needs. She plans light, nutritious meals and collects recipes with friends to make her cooking activities more enjoyable. She dresses only in clothes she feels comfortable in. She takes weekends away with friends several times per year. She takes daily walks with her husband, and the children join them when they're home to do so. She sets aside an inviolate time for study and reading (which also helps the children create their own inviolate study time). She attends a woman's reading group. She goes bicycle riding frequently with her family or other neighborhood women. When she needs household products, she tries to buy ones that make her feel pampered, such as soaps with favorite scents. And, much to her own surprise, because she's always seen herself as wanting to have a "natural look," she now lightens her hair color, which for her turned out to be the most symbolically important aspect of her reclaiming her femininity and attractiveness.

The key for her is that she really listened carefully to the inner signals that directed her toward replenishing activities. She let go of preconceived judgments about what "should" make her feel replenished. She decided she was important enough to give these things to herself. Indeed, her success at this endeavor is evident, as she is a person whose countenance has a glow that is with her wherever she goes. She doesn't forget her encounter with cancer; she has turned it around to make a richer, more vital and balanced life.

UNITY

We cannot separate human life from the body. All our experiences in this world—sights, sounds, smells, tastes, touch, vibes, auras, intuition, simple and complex feeling of all kinds, our sense of time and place, what we perceive and what we ignore—are brought to us in their initial form courtesy of our physical selves. Our bodies are terrific sending and receiving devices in the circular exchange of information with the environment and with others. They are also as much the repository of experience as are the realms of the mind or feelings. From the most material to the most symbolic, the overt to the implicate, we are what we experience (Kaschak 1992).

In Western thinking, the mind, spirit (or soul), and body are seen as separate and separable entities. This view survives despite considerable evidence, including scientific evidence, of the connections among these aspects of self that cannot be unraveled from each other. Further, Westerners usually describe themselves as *having* a body or a mind or a spirit rather than *being* a body or a mind or a spirit. We are thus lead to believe that we *own or possess* a body, a mind, and a spirit. It is probably much more accurate to conceive of ourselves as *being* an "embodied-mindful-spirited" creature of the earth. Further, it probably means something slightly different to each woman to think of herself as a *female* embodied-mindful-spirited creature.

Our **body** transports us around. It gives us the medium to send out and take in all sorts of information, and thus to have experiences. The ability to send and receive authentically useful information is often a maturing force over our lifetimes. Our **psyche** is another name for our place of experience of emotions. Our emotions are meant to be strong, useful, reactive and proactive signals to help us come to conclusions about what we are experiencing. To move from a blaming position to a position of self-responsibility is to mature the emotions, the psyche. To balance the existential drives to be self-directed with the unchangeable "givens" of your particular life is also to mature the psyche. Our **mind** might be another name for our brain. This is our place or experience of thinking, recognizing, understanding, planning, learning, attitudes, deciding. To mature the mind is to keep all these activities in reasonable balance with each other, as they are all very useful. Our **soul** or spirit is often called things such as the place or experience of beauty, peace, finding the self, a higher power, spirituality, infinity, nature valuation, and wisdom. The maturing of the soul is to be in the active process of searching, searching for meaningfulness and purpose.

All of these "parts" of ourselves are not really separable parts at all. They are more *ways to express* our many different means of experiencing ourselves and our worlds. And again, these experiential processes may have unique meaning for each woman, if she were to consider what it means to her to be a female body, a female psyche, a female mind, and a female soul. Some of these aspects may "feel" more or less feminine to her. In some aspects, the traditional female stereotypes may be more ingrained and therefore call for more reconsideration than in others. Some of these aspects may seem to have more overlap with each other than do others.

A diagnosis of breast cancer or gynecologic cancer can at first obscure all these wonderful faculties and aspects of experience that are at our service. As we begin to emerge from initial, emergency, survival modes, the awareness of these unified faculties can again begin to make their dynamic balances known. And many women find that it becomes important to them to make these dynamic balances on a more aware and awake basis than they may have done formerly.

An inspiring example of living as a balanced embodied-mindful-spirited creature is seen in another patient of mine.

This woman had a combination of uterine cancer and colon disease that resulted in surgery to remove her reproductive organs plus the creation of an artificial diversionary opening for her colon, called a colostomy, which meant that the digestive fecal matter was diverted to empty from her body via an opening created in her abdomen instead of from the usual anal opening. Ostomies to collect the stool require the use of a special bag that is strapped to the body and emptied regularly by the patient herself. This woman had previously been very active as an athlete, and at first she felt that her ostomy would make her life completely sedentary.

A turning point came when her husband was able to convey to her that he still saw her as feminine and attractive despite the new apparatus. From his view, she was able to begin remaking her own new view of femininity that included her former sense of athletic strength. She decided she would have to change to different forms of athleticism, so she took up the study of yoga. In yoga she found a method of dedicating herself to building several important traits that were central to her values: physical strength and emotional strength, physical flexibility and emotional flexibility, and a spiritual path that integrated body, mind, and spirit. The competencies that were inspired by her yoga practice further helped her find renewed avenues for other ways to enhance her quality of life, and she took up basketball coaching at the local high school where her grandchildren attended. Also, she and her husband became avid gardeners, tending both the gardens and their relationship at the same time. Like so many cancer patients, she first mourned her losses and changes, then she turned her life around to make an integrated, balanced wholeness out of her new circumstances.

HEARING OUR OWN VOICE

As children in a Western culture, young women are discouraged from speaking fully and intensely about feelings, real selves, and loves and hates. This in turn cuts away our ability to experience our lives with gusto. Our wildness, our opinions and feelings, our subjective experience are all devalued and asked to stay underground—precisely because of their emotional powerfulness. In the stoic Western cultures, powerfully expressed feelings are discouraged. We live in a society that fears and pathologizes feelings (Bepko and Krestan 1993). When we are not encouraged to feel our opinions and emotions and are not encouraged to express them and practice them, it becomes most difficult to use them wisely and to modulate their useful expression. This also can result in a self-alienation, in a silencing of the self, in a belief that others are full of value while oneself is of low worth. The further result can be obsessiveness, depression, creating vicious circles, and addictions. Obsessions and addictions are often seen as attempted solutions to the lack of connection with oneself. Depression is often the reaction to this lack of self-connection. When one feels worthless, one seeks the love and approval of others to give oneself value. This is value-by-association with a valued person rather than a real, internal awareness of self value.

When a woman with cancer listens well to her own inner voice, she can often hear what it is among all these stereotypes, abilities, acuities, traits, and aspects that is amiss. From a woman's frame of reference, there are ways to describe that something is wrong that we realize are familiar experiences, but we may never have had words put to them. These experiences, these inner voices, often need to be translated from their first, impressionistic, inchoate forms into recognizable language in order to understand them more fully ourselves and to communicate with others.

These impression-voices, as described by Estés (1992), might be signals such as feeling extraordinarily dry, fatigued, frail, depressed, confused, gagged, muzzled, frightened, without inspiration, without animation, without soulfulness, without meaning, chronically fuming, stuck, volatile, uncreative, powerless, chronically doubtful, blocked, giving one's creative life over to others, overprotective of oneself, inert, unable to pace oneself or set limits, not insistent on one's own tempo, to be far from one's god(s), to fear to venture by oneself, to fear to reveal oneself, fearful to set out one's imperfect work before it is an opus, wincing, or having humiliation, angst, numbness, anxiety. It is as if we have had a strong voice within ourselves all along, but we often have to make an extra effort to hear it if its volume has been tuned low because of unsavory childhood experiences or traumatic events or cultural messages and beliefs.

One patient I remember came to see me at the point in her life where she had grown tired of so often feeling these subliminal sensations of everything being amiss—she said she had felt pressured and trapped and empty and uncreative and powerless for as long as she could remember, and it was just dawning on her that these might be signals not of some "truth" about her life but signals of a need to make some changes instead. The catalyst had been a recent diagnosis of breast cancer. As she was recovering from her surgeries and treatments, she'd had one of those "Aha!" experiences, a voice within that said she certainly did not want to return to her former life that had consisted of working far too many hours, a stormy and unsatisfying marriage, lack of involvement with her child, and no social and leisure outlets.

Her first step, after listening to her own voice and recognizing these important inner messages, was to build a belief in herself that she was capable of constructing a better life. Next, she had to figure out what her own definition of a better life might be. It was my privilege as her therapist to help her with these tasks and to be able to watch her blossom. It took awhile, but she was able to set clearer boundaries at her job, which allowed her to work fewer hours and yet feel better about what she did contribute to the company. She eventually left her marriage and is allowing herself to search for a partner who makes a better match for her. She began to volunteer at her daughter's school to add to her involvement with her daughter's life. And even though her time is limited, as a single mother, she chose to take classes in beadwork, where she could feel creative and also meet some social needs. She says there is more she wants to do to keep enhancing her life, but she also knows she is someone who fares best when she takes things slowly.

Women's cancer, like nothing else, can help us hear these useful voices again so that we may recognize what is amiss—and especially so that we can begin to fix it. These feelings and inner voices are precisely meant for the purpose of aiding our understanding of what might be wrong and what we might do to mend it.

Women's cancer, like nothing else, can become the catalyst to fully see the many aspects of ourselves, to reevaluate our values and priorities. To do so lays the foundation for living an enriched, choiceful, redecided life that is based on new and amended definitions of womanhood—and of humanness.

2

The Cancers
of Women

Children growing up in the American Southwest, drinking contaminated milk from contaminated cows, even
from the contaminated breasts of their mothers, my
mother—members, years later, of the Clan of One-
Breasted Women. . . . One by one, I have watched the
women in my family die common, heroic deaths. We sat
in waiting rooms hoping for good news, but always receiving the bad. I cared for them, bathed their scarred bodies,
and kept their secrets. I watched beautiful women become
bald as Cytoxan, cisplatin, and Adriamycin were injected
into their veins. I held their foreheads as they vomited
green-black bile, and I shot them with morphine when the
pain became inhuman. In the end, I witnessed their last
peaceful breaths, becoming a midwife to the rebirth of

their souls. I cannot prove that my mother, Diane Dixon
Tempest, or my grandmothers, Lettie Romney Dixon and
Kathryn Blackett Tempest, along with my aunts developed
cancer from nuclear fallout in Utah. But I can't prove they
didn't. [Williams 1991]

Women experience women's cancers in very deep and
personal ways. We are complex creatures, full of symbolic
references, conscious and subconscious, that drive our experience of ourselves. This is especially true in our experience of our own womanhood or femininity. It is useful to
attend to these meanings for ourselves; doing so is a good
aid to living richly, despite limitations.

When we first hear our diagnosis, we are often blind-
sided by our own associations with the word cancer, plus
our personal associations about the organs involved. At this
particularly difficult time, we also are bombarded with a lot
of never-before-heard medical terminology, the treatment
options, and even the blame! "Nice girls and repressed
women get cancer" (you never got angry enough, after being
told all your life never to get angry), or "over-sexed women
reap what they sow" (the belief that promiscuous sexual
activity is related to pelvic cancers), or my personal un-
favorite, "women who get breast cancer needed to get something 'off their chest'" (Give me a break!). There is so much
to sort out early in the cancer experience.

The "Cancer Personality" that some sources describe
fits everyone and therefore no one. It also connotes a lot
of negatives: someone who gives too much, doesn't laugh
enough, is too angry or alternately isn't angry enough, is
suppressed, doesn't express emotions, has poor relation-

ships, and doesn't eat proper foods. This description fits plenty of people *without* cancer. And it is quite undescriptive of plenty of women who have had cancer. This also fails to encourage us, cancer patients and nonpatients alike, occasionally to reevaluate our lives in terms of both its "blessings and curses" (Rose 1995). Blaming ourselves is a very different approach than taking rightful responsibility.

There is no real evidence of any personality style or emotional traits associated with cancers. Studies show that cancer patients did not have any greater life stressors before their cancer than did women without cancer. Also, these studies show that women who have a recurrence of their cancer have not been under more stress than are women who do not have a recurrence. There is also no relationship between a woman's level of psychological adjustment and the severity of her cancer (Atkinson 1994). Rather, cancers are substantially more likely to be associated with exposure to unseen environmental toxins, substances ingested early in life before you were old enough to study the quality of your food, genetic predisposition, or a complex interplay of hormonal and other biological factors that we know much too little about. You can make choices about some of these factors from now on, and it can feel very healthy and right to make these choices, but you are still faced with some level of unknown causes and an unknown future. Here lies the difficult but exhilarating existential task of making a renewed life.

Much of the coverage of women's cancers presented by television and magazine media gives the impression that cancer is little more than a fashion and lifestyle bummer. You might lose your breast or your uterus or your hair and become just a little less productive on your job for a week or two, but after you've had surgeries for the requisite replacement of missing organs, your hair will grow back and you'll look just fine again. It's hard to come to grips with the cold fact that you have what is essentially an incurable disease, a disease that despite three decades of intense funding still leaves the medical field nearly clueless about how to prevent these cancers and save our lives (Hooper 1994). To take the position that cancer is just a cosmetic event is to be deeply robbed of the real meanings that the disease has for you and to miss the chance to live the remainder of your life from a full reevaluated and reprioritized position.

Many women experience their cancer diagnosis first and foremost as a threat. The threats can be multiple, including a threat to her sense of self, to her body's integrity, to her lifestyle and activities, to her dreams, and to relationships. Further, she may feel the threat of feared pain, of disfigurement and dismemberment, of loss of work, of loss of opportunities, of being a burden, of dependency, of depression. Indeed, she may have to think hard about the threatening meaning of no longer being able to perceive herself as a fully healthy person, at least not for a while, or perhaps not ever. She may be faced with the threat of lost body parts or loss of normal bodily function, such as bowel or bladder function, or sexual function, as she has known them in the past. Also, many women are threatened by the fear that their disease will make them less respected or less loved, and that they might therefore lose the closeness of loved ones.

Beyond the experience of threat, women begin to view their cancer from many possible perspectives. Some may see their cancer as a challenge to be overcome or a problem to be solved. Some experience it as an enemy or a punishment, and women with pelvic and breast cancers may be particularly vulnerable to the inaccurate belief that their cancer is a consequence of past sexual transgressions. Some women experience their cancer as a relief—from responsibilities or demands that they have been unable to find a way to refuse in the past. Some women experience it simply as an irreparable loss, and from this view can come either a feeling of inferiority because of having to live what may be an impaired life, or a feeling of healthy grief that first mourns the losses and then regathers itself to create a renewed outlook on life. Finally, some women experience their cancer as an event with positive aspects, perhaps helping a woman view her life with more appreciation, more meaning, more value. Probably, part or all of these views are present and are meant to be wrestled with. Most of us realize early on that we will never be the same again.

Also, a woman's age at the time of diagnosis may contribute to her unique responses to her cancer. For example, a young adult woman may be in a developmental stage where she still carries some vestiges of the adolescent's extreme sensitivity to any disease process that could affect her appearance. Also, in young adulthood, many women still experience a sense of invulnerability; this could either be an aid in helping her bounce back from treatments and fearful states or a detriment in contributing to denial or lack of followthrough with treatments.

In contrast, a woman in her thirties or forties could experience her cancer in the context of the psychological-developmental tasks of that age, which are to establish a niche for her life and balance her ability to give to others while nurturing herself. At this age, women may be confronted with a difficulty in receiving or asking for the care she needs, both physical and emotional. Or at one end of a continuum, she could feel energized to make sure her own values and purposes in life are met—now that her time may feel shortened—while at the other end of this continuum, she could feel thwarted from being able to carry out her life dreams.

For women in their fifties or sixties or so, the developmental tasks that are in the foreground relate to an emphasis on continued balance of needs and a creation of personally satisfying movement into older adulthood. In these ages, a woman's diagnosis of cancer may bear particular meaning on her sense of having a future. It may also make an impression on her view of the effect of her own history so far, thus having either a positive or negative effect on her sense of efficacy, that is, on her belief in herself to take as much charge of her life as is available given the cards she has been dealt.

A woman in her mid-sixties or seventies and better often enters a stage of psychological development that emphasizes a sense of generativity, that is, a knowledge of what legacy she may be able to leave behind her while continuing to maintain a satisfactory level of activity and purpose in her life. Here, a diagnosis of cancer may take on a meaning that relates to her sense of accomplishment and of betterment— of her world and of herself.

A woman with children may experience yet further singular meanings about her cancer diagnosis. These meanings, and feelings, will often be colored by the age and abilities of the children, the quality of the family, the quality of nearby caregivers, and satisfaction with who might serve as a good mothering figure when she is not able to do so herself, either through times of illness or after her death. Further, effects of diagnosis can be influenced by how willing the mother herself is to be able to be a good role model to her children, a role model of showing honest feelings and reactions, of balanced giving and receiving, and of a graceful or meaningful acceptance she can provide of one's unwanted stumbling stones in life.

The word cancer often conjures twin meanings. First, it is seen as a tumor, a terrible and deforming disease. Second, cancer is often a judgment, replete with recoiling and fear, an indication of lack of vitality. The woman with a newly diagnosed cancer—and her loved ones as well—are often faced with making new meanings out of these associations. In chapter 1, I described the responses from a group of women whom I asked to give their associations to the words "womanhood" and "femininity." These same women listed the following terms in response to the word *cancer*. In descending order of frequency, the word cancer brought to mind the ideas of *fear, suffering, dread, loss of control over one's life, hurt, danger, pain, disfigurement, reevaluation of life, eating away, lack of self care, sadness, eating from inside, wild cells, growths, destruction, breasts, wasting away, loss, despair, scary, "it won't happen to me," terror, facing death, rot, "changed my life," "I hope I don't get it again," robber, evil,* and *"do I have it?"* Clearly, it can be an enhancing and cleansing activity to find each of our own personal lists such as this so that we may fully comprehend cancer's meanings to us. Doing so helps us see its power and tangle with that power; if you have a dragon to fight, it really helps if you can see the dragon and know its traits and its power. This gives you strategy advantage.

WOMEN AND THE WORLD OF MEDICINE

It may be surprising to learn that in the field of psychology, it is only in the last two or three decades that it has been recognized that the study of *women's psychology* should be an area of special attention. Previous to that time, nearly all volunteers and paid subjects in psychological research had been males, nearly all theories had been based on males as the norm, and, notably, mostly women, not men, had been studied as "case material" for examples of neuroticism and ineffective living. Thus, empirical literature in psychology often bears several biases. Not only may solely male subjects be used in the experiment, but the researchers may not test for sex differences, they may build theories by eliminating data from females that do not correspond to data from males, they may lack knowledge of sex roles and how these roles may influence behavior in the experiment, and they may use predominantly male experimenters. Also, in psychological literature it is common to view behaviors as dichotomous rather than integrated, especially conceptualizing masculinity and femininity as mutually exclusive and contradictory of each other rather than as overlapping concepts (Kaschak 1992).

Perhaps it is even more surprising to learn that in the field of medicine, it is only in the last one or two decades that the study of *women's health* has been recognized as an area in need of special attention. Until very recently, the selection and definition of problems for study, the exclusion of females as experimental subjects, a bias in the methodology used to collect and interpret data, and bias in the theories and conclusions drawn from the data in clinical trials often failed to include women or women's changing needs through the life span. This has given rise to potential distortion in understanding risk factors and in determining which treatments are best for each gender. Further, because the practice of modern medicine depends heavily on clinical research, any flaws, deletions, and ethical problems in this research are likely to result in poorer health care and inequity in the medical treatment of disadvantaged groups—anyone who is not a white, middle- to upper-class male. The choice of problems for study is determined by funding, which in turn is largely in control of the members of the U. S. Congress and of federal agencies such as the National Institutes of Health. Both of these institutional bodies consist of mostly white middle- to upper-class males.

Further, nearly all research that has so far been conducted on women's health has focused on only two areas: procreation and heterosexual activity. This state of affairs shows that so far, women's health care has only been defined in terms of women's relationships with men. There is very little research on matters of high medical importance to women themselves, including breast and gynecological cancers, eating disorders, dysmenorrhea (painful or extremely heavy menstrual periods), lesbian health care, pelvic inflammatory disease, osteoporosis, and incontinence and hip fractures in elderly women.

Having a preponderance of white males setting the priorities for medical research results in research that certainly is not formulated to focus on gender. This is especially a problem where gender differences exist in the frequency of diseases, the symptoms of diseases, responses to treatments, or the complications of diseases. This means that when exploring the metabolism of a particular drug, tests may be run only on males and not on females. This may include the tests run on your chemotherapy agent, for example. These types of bias raise ethical, and personal, issues: Health care practitioners must treat the majority of the population, which is female (yes, there are more women in the world than men), based on information gathered from clinical research in which drugs may not have been tested on females, in which the cause and course of the disease in women has not been studied, and in which women's experience has been ignored (Rosser 1994).

As of this writing, just over 40% of medical students now are women, a change from 28 years ago in 1970, when the number was only 10%. However, women remain concentrated in the fields of general medicine, pediatrics, and psychiatry, but our numbers are increasing noticeably in residencies in all specialties. This signals a dramatic change in the composition of practicing physicians, which may in turn have an impact on attention to women's health issues outside of the research arena.

In 1990 (at long last!) the Office of Research on Women's Health was established at the National Institutes of Health in the U.S. The purpose of the Office was to address the previous underrepresentation of women in medical studies. Some impact has been seen so far not only in an increased number of women included in medical outcome studies but in including women of color rather than recruiting mostly Caucasian subjects. It is these studies that have brought us some of the following preliminary and useful information (*Harvard Women's Health Watch* 1996): for women, health benefits do result from regular exercise, eating fresh fruits and vegetables, and maintaining a lean body mass; taking estrogen alone (without other hormones) after menopause is associated with the occurrence of endometrial (uterine) cancer; drinking alcohol is associated with increased incidence of breast cancer (three alcoholic drinks per week is thought to be a cut-off); and sunbathing is associated with increased incidence of melanoma. Current studies from this Office are looking at the degree to which taking hormone replacements after menopause lowers the risk of heart disease and of osteoporosis but increases the risk of breast and gynecological cancers; whether estrogen has an effect on staying mentally sharp into older ages; and a study of the physical and psychological differences among African-American, Hispanic, Asian-American, and Caucasian women during menopause.

Health information about, and outreach to, minority women population groups is an especially needed area of redress and is just barely getting off the ground. The reasons usually cited for lower utilization of health care among ethnic minority and sexual minority women include fear of discrimination, lack of money, lack of health insurance, distrust of health care providers, and lack of accurate information about the need for health care and the risk factors for disease. These are large hurdles to overcome and probably do not comprise the whole picture, but some national and local research is underway to illuminate these specialty issues.

We do have some preliminary information available and can make a few educated guesses as well. For instance, it is believed that lesbians have a much lower incidence of cervical cancer than non-lesbian women do (as well as a lower incidence of many sexually transmitted diseases). These lower rates may be related to lower frequency of heterosexual sexual activity. In contrast, lesbians are presently thought to be at higher risk for breast and uterine cancers, although the data so far are not very conclusive. If there is a higher incidence of these cancers, it is speculated to be because of one or more factors that are possible risk factors for women's cancers: First, it is believed that fewer lesbians have children than heterosexual women, and lack of pregnancies before the age of 30 is a probable cancer risk factor; second, women with higher body fat are at higher risk, and overweight conditions are more acceptable in some segments of the lesbian community; third, because of the need for Pap smears in order to receive birth control pills, heterosexual women go to a physician more frequently than do lesbians, and thus lesbian women are also encouraged less or referred less often for mammograms, breast examinations, and pelvic examinations that can detect early cancers; fourth, many lesbians are hindered from seeking health care due to feared homophobia and insensitivity on the part of health care practitioners; fifth, although most lesbians view their lesbianism as a positive force in their lives, many also note that being a lesbian in a homophobic society is quite stressful, perhaps even more so for lesbians of color. Stress may well have a role in many disease processes, including cardiovascular disease, gastrointestinal problems, lupus erythematosis, and skin allergies.

There will be a twofold perennial problem in studying risk factors and providing information to lesbian populations. One is that the stigma against homosexuality will make many women unwilling to state the real depth of their relationship with another woman; such women would certainly not be likely to volunteer for any medical or psychological research designated as looking for lesbian subjects. Also, many women who love a woman in a partnership do not define that relationship as "lesbian," although it may be a long-term, loving, committed relationship. These women also would not appear among possible research subjects in lesbian-identified protocols.

For minority groups in general, both lesbians and women of color, health care access may be hindered by economic factors as well as the possibility of discrimination. While it is certainly not universally so, statistically more minority women may find it financially prohibitive to obtain recommended health care screening on a regular basis. Minority women in the U.S.—both ethnic minorities and sexual minorities—are proportionately more likely to be without health insurance coverage due to marginal employment or to the absence of a male contributor to the household finances or less likely to have insurance coverage through a spouse.

Further, the common avenues of information of medical information may not be as readily available to minority women. Community health efforts are necessary to increase cancer screening programs, stop smoking programs, exercise, weight loss, and alcohol programs directed especially for minority women, since smoking, obesity, and alcohol consumption are among the risk factors for cancer. Also, alcohol consumption is found to be higher among minority, oppressed populations in the U.S. Poor Caucasian women, of course, face similar obstacles.

At this time, much too little is known about the risk factors that may apply to different populations of women: ethnic minorities, lesbians, or women in poverty, for instance. This information would be useful in that it would allow community health projects to prioritize areas of public health concern (Bowen 1994). Efforts are just now beginning around the country to learn more about the cancer risk factors for different populations. We know, for instance that African-American women in the U.S. experience a lower frequency of breast cancer but also experience lower survival rates when they do get breast cancer compared with Caucasian women. As this type of information becomes available, it can be combined with understanding of the sociocultural factors that affect health-related behaviors to design interventions aimed at behavior changes and cancer prevention in specific populations.

HOW CANCER HAPPENS

Cancers are a group of related diseases in which cells of a particular tissue type become abnormal and divide. The cells do not respond to normal control mechanisms, and they grow in a disorderly fashion. They invade and damage nearby tissue and organs. When these cancers break away from the original tumor, they may enter the bloodstream or lymph system and circulate throughout the body. This gives the cancer cells an opportunity to spread to other sites, establish themselves, and subsequently grow in other parts of the body, forming a metastasis. It is this spreading, or metastatic process (see Figure 1), that eventually effects a large enough amount of body tissue, causing death by using the body's energy stores and by inhibiting the activity of normal and vital organs. Because cancers can take many years to grow to a size where they can be felt, pinpointing just when or where a metastasis might be likely to take hold is very difficult. We can only predict possible sites and timing based on the experience of women with cancer who have forged the paths ahead of us.

Part of the increase in breast and gynecologic cancers results from the boring fact that cancer is more likely in older people, and more women are now living to older ages than in previous human history. The very fact of senescence, of aging, means that the environment of any cell and its regulatory capabilities are deteriorating.

More interesting is that the probability of a cancer of the female reproductive system at any age appears to increase directly in relation to the number of menstrual cycles a

The primary cancer forms a tumor nodule.

The tumor breaks through its limiting membrane and invades other tissue in the primary organ site.

Tumor clumps invade blood vessels and lymphatic vessels, float in the blood or lymph in the vessel, adhere to the vessel wall downstream, and penetrate the vessel to migrate out into tissue at another site where a tumor grows again and forms a metastasis at a site distant from the primary tumor.

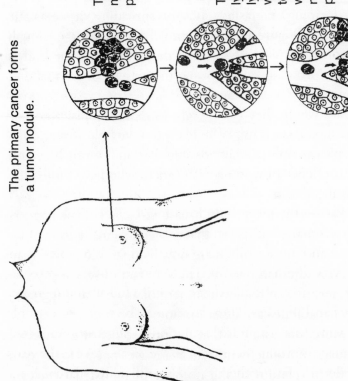

FIGURE 1. The Metastatic Process

woman has experienced. The most likely host of a cancer of the reproductive tissues is an elderly woman who had an early menarche (first period) and a late menopause and never had her cycling interrupted by pregnancy and lactation (breastfeeding). The Stone Age woman, to whom we are still evolutionarily and physically nearly identical, had a very different sort of reproductive life history than does the modern day woman. Perhaps because she was less well nourished and more heavily laden with bacteria or parasites, she started menstrual periods much later and experienced menopause much earlier. (These are probably the same reasons that her overall life expectancy was shorter than ours: She most likely died of malnutrition and infection, while women in our time die of cancers and heart disease.)

Further, Stone Age woman was frequently pregnant, with lactation usually carried out for 2 to 4 years after each birth, which is associated with inhibition of the menstrual cycle. Her average age of death was about 45. In her 25 to 30 reproductive years, she would have been pregnant or lactating approximately half the time, and her total number of menstrual cycles could not have been much more than 150. A modern woman, even if she has two or three children, will likely experience the hormonal washings of the menstrual cycle somewhere in the neighborhood of 375 times! Further, it is theorized that breast tissue and other reproductive tissues may not fully develop until a full-term pregnancy occurs and that immature tissue may be more susceptible to carcinogens. The initial mutations that set women's cancers in motion may occur prior to age 35 and take many years to manifest. Researchers could be diligently searching for means to mimic the low cancer rates that come naturally to women in hunter-gatherer societies. This does not preclude searching just as diligently for other environmental, dietary, and genetic causes of cancer (Nesse and Williams 1994).

For a cancer to form, it must navigate an amazing obstacle course of safeguards. First, it must have a breakdown in its encoded message to stop growing when it is mature so that it continues to grow anyway. That is, it must escape the DNA "editing and repair" that is built into cell life, a feat that may result from genetic disposition, environmental interference, injuries, illnesses, nutritional or metabolic states, or simply the reduced efficiency of cellular regulatory mechanisms that comes with aging. The cancer cell must also escape the inhibitory effect of tumor suppresser genes. (One such gene, called p53, was recently discovered to make a protein that protects against cancer by regulating the expression of other genes that are misbehaving. The gene is found to be abnormal in 40 percent of breast cancers studied.) Finally, there is the immune system, with its host of weapons designed to identify and minimize maladaptive growth as soon as it finds a difference between it and normal growth. A detectable cancer must achieve the improbable feat of getting through these many layers of defense.

But looked at another way, we probably have dozens to hundreds of misbehaving cells appearing every day, given the 10 trillion cells that comprise the human body. From this point of view, what is amazing is that we get so *few* cancers, because what cancer has on its side is the astronomical number of chances it gets to achieve success against immense odds. Cancer is entirely the product of chance alterations in the cellular regulatory machinery (Nesse and Williams 1994).

> I have a theory about cancer cell. I do not think they
> are evil in the sense that Hitler was evil. They are
> simply buffoons, cells so dumb they can't even tran-
> scribe the DNA message right. [Hooper, 1994]

The Quality Control Inspector breaks down in cancer's development. The inspector is allowing a cell with damaged DNA (whether damaged by pesticides, hormones, genetic programming, diet, lifestyle, or other things we do not know yet) to divide and grow—it's supposed to note the damage and allow the cell to die. Research studying ways of fixing what breaks down the Inspector's vigilance is ongoing and will hopefully be given even more attention in the future. Perhaps someday anti-angiogenesis drugs may be figured out, which would block cancer cells from obtaining the blood supply they need to grow and spread. Inventing bigger and better chemotherapy, radiation, and toxic drug treatments likely are not the only answers. However, currently, the toxic treatments and surgeries are our best-known survival tools.

Do you recall your high school biology class lesson on cell division? Like any cell, a cancer cell starts out as just one cell. It takes roughly 90 days for this cell to divide and become two cells. In another 90 days or so, these will have divided and become 4 cells. Ninety days more and the group becomes 8 cells. If you keep counting this out, you'll see that it can take a whole year for the cancer tumor to get to just 16 cells. This is way too small to feel. But it might be visible after another several multiplications on a particularly good mammogram. It is believed that by the time a breast cancer is large enough to feel with your fingers, about the size of a pea, the cancer has been around for several years, perhaps as many as 9 or 10.

Also, it's not the cancerous tumor you can feel as a lump, it's the nearby cells reacting to the cancer. Some cancers never went through this arithmetical growth and don't cause any reaction until they are quite large. Pelvic cancers also, then, are often not findable until they are many years old and big enough to cause functional problems or pain from pressing on nearby organs. The good news about this is that you can take a little extra time to make your treatment decisions—you don't have to decide them all today. This is especially good since most of us humans have a *first reaction* that says one thing but a *considered reaction* that may guide us in another direction.

Doctors used to think that these cancers began in the primary organ, such as breast or ovary or uterus, and got out into the rest of the body via the lymph system. But we now know that blood vessels growing into the primary tumor appear by year 2, and currently, cancers often aren't treated until they are found at about year 10. Certainly, some cancerous cells have gotten out by then via the blood circulatory system, if not the lymph system as well. This is why, even if the lymph nodes you had removed during surgery have no sign of cancer ("negative lymph nodes"), a metastasis elsewhere in the body will still show up about 30% of the time. Conversely, if your lymph nodes did have cancer in them ("positive lymph nodes"), there is approximately a 60% chance of metastasis, not 100%.

But given how long this cancer has already been in your body, and the possibility of stray cancer cells migrating around the body through either the blood or lymph systems, why has it not spread to other parts of the body any more than it has? The answer is your immune system. An immune system that is in tip-top shape can probably handle all the little stray cancer cells that may appear in our bodies every day and may also be able to take care of any stray cells that are breaking off from a known tumor. The best cancer prevention we know of so far is a well-running immune system.

The many cancer patients I have seen in my office over the years all seem to want to find a cause for their cancer. This makes utter sense to me, as our brains are hard-wired to organize, understand, and seek causes and explanations for all our experiences. Not only do our brains drive this desire to find a cause, but so do our souls, I believe. So, brain and soul can go on a journey of discovery to make *personal* sense out of the cancer, and I indeed encourage my patients to do this. But I encourage each woman to make her own meaning of her cancer. Our brain piece may want to know medical and statistical information, like how cells can go awry, but our soul piece seeks information that isn't factual but instead is personally formed to make sense of the *way* in which we are experiencing and responding to this soul-shaking earthquake we call cancer. Some women conclude that their cancer is clearly a random cellular fact or a genetic happenstance, some conclude it's their diet or behavior or activities, some conclude it's exposure to toxins, still others attribute it to stress or bad circumstances. The point is not to find which answer is *right*, but to find answers you can live with. Often, these personal conclusions that we choose can become helpful guides for more optimal living in the future.

THE DIAGNOSIS

The diagnosis of a woman's cancer leaves many women and their loved ones in a mind-boggling, disorienting state of being overwhelmed. The medical information and treatment descriptions can come across as so much mumbo jumbo as to defy understanding. When we are in a state of emergency, as often happens right after hearing the diagnosis, it may take several explanations before we grasp the difference between, for instance, chemotherapy and radiation. However, most of what a woman needs to know is quite understandable and quite explainable. And I believe strongly that the more she knows, the more a woman can come to terms with her choices, her actions, her waves of emotional states, and her treatment effects. That is, if she has lots and lots of information, she will be able to make decisions, to understand and work with her own reactions, and to ask for what she needs in ways that feel authentic.

More importantly, some of the decisions we are faced with have no certain outcomes. Medical studies (and psychological studies, too) by their very nature address volumes of people, and precise, individual predictions are not very possible in all cases. Also, humans are so complex that it is again nearly infeasible to completely understand the role of every possible factor contributing to our health or to our response to a treatment. This is a very difficult situation to be in, and one of the best things we can do for ourselves is to ensure that in the future we will be able to know we made reasonably good decisions at this time based on reasonably abundant information—because doing so leaves little room for deep regret or dissatisfaction. A woman will then always be able to look back at this time and say she was as thorough as she could reasonably be and that she made decisions based on the breadth of information available to her at the time.

So, explaining and often reexplaining any and all information a woman wants is one of the most helpful things that a loved one or medical or psychological professional can do. Here, I will review much of the information—medical and statistical information and experiences of women with cancers themselves—that cancer patients may find useful and empowering, whether they are recently diagnosed or have their cancer many years behind them.

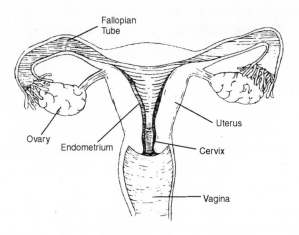

FIGURE 2. Front View of the Reproductive Organs

For many women, knowing they are not alone, knowing how many women share their experience, is useful, so let's start with the "numbers", gathered from yearly compilations published in the journal *CA* (Parker et al. 1996, 1997). Each year, approximately 185,000 new breast cancers and 82,000 new pelvic cancers are diagnosed. Of all cancers diagnosed in women per year, 30% are breast cancer, 6% are uterine cancer, 4% are ovarian cancer, and 2% are cervical cancer. And each year, approximately 44,000 women die of their breast cancer and 26,500 die of their pelvic cancer. Of all cancer deaths per year, 17% of deaths are from breast cancer, 5% from ovarian cancer, and 2% each are from cervical and uterine cancers for women of all races combined. (Lung cancer kills more women than any other cancer: 25% of cancer deaths over the life span. However, breast and pelvic cancers kill more *young* women [ages 15–55] than does lung cancer.)

Some differences in cancer rates do exist by race and ethnicity. Of all deaths from cancer in the United States, approximately 8% of deaths are from breast cancer among Caucasian, African-American, and Hispanic women; 6% are among Native Americans, Asians and Pacific Islanders. For ovarian cancer, approximately 2.5% of cancer deaths per year occur among Caucasian, Native American, and Hispanic women; for African-American, Asian, and Pacific Islander women, ovarian cancer accounts for less than 2% of cancer deaths. The differences in these comparative percentages are small, but the actual numbers of women's lives that they represent are notable.

The 1996 statistics on African-American women show the following: breast cancer deaths numbered 5,200; cervical cancer deaths, 3,360; uterine cancer deaths, 1,100; and ovarian cancer deaths, 940. Breast cancer continues to be the second leading cause of death from cancers for African-American women; only lung cancer causes more deaths, although these numbers are not very disparate (5,200 deaths to breast cancer in 1996 compared to 5,900 deaths to lung cancer). The mortality rate for African-American women exceeds the mortality rate for Caucasian women for breast cancer and for all gynecological cancers. The same is true for Hispanic women, although not as much as for African-Americans.

New cancer cases estimated for 1996 for African-American women are as follows: breast cancer, 16,600; cervical cancer, 2,300; uterine cancer, 2,100; ovarian cancer, 1,700. Breast cancer constitutes the highest rate of new diagnoses among all cancers for these women. Cervical cancers are diagnosed in African-American women at 1.7 times the rate of diagnosis in Caucasian women, but the rates of discovery and diagnosis do not otherwise differ notably among these two groups. Cancers of the breast and pelvic organs are more often found at a later stage or when a distant metastasis is already present than is true for Caucasian women.

Our knowledge so far of genetic aspects of cancers is also beneficial to many women. Studies of families with inherited alterations in the BRCA 1 gene or BRCA 2 gene (BR stands for breast, CA stands for cancer) suggest that more than half of women who carry a cancer-associated mutation in the gene will be diagnosed with breast cancer by age 50, and as many as 85% to 90% (some studies say even more) will be diagnosed by age 70 (*Coping* 1995 Sept./Oct.; Bowen 1994). These studies also indicate that as much as 44% of women with mutations of the BRCA genes will get ovarian cancer. It is estimated that women in these very high risk families, however, make up only a very small percentage of women who get cancer; some studies indicate only 1% to 4% of breast cancer cases are related to these mutations, and other studies indicate that 6% to 10% of all breast cancer cases are related to the mutations. Either way, familial genetic circumstances are definitely not the most common cause of breast cancers. Other gynecologic cancers may also be associated with these genetic alterations, but less is known about this yet.

Very recent studies indicate that these high risk numbers may be misleading and may only apply to a certain population of women with BRCA gene mutations. The 85% risk for breast cancer and 44% risk for ovarian cancer may only be relevant for women of Eastern Jewish descent who have family members who have also been diagnosed with these cancers. For women whose family members are mostly cancer-free, the risk may be closer to 55% for breast cancer by age 70 and 16% for ovarian cancer by age 70. So far, nearly all of this research has been conducted with Jewish women, and its extrapolation to other women is still unknown.

The research indicates that these inherited mutations do not cause breast cancer themselves. Rather, a tumor can begin to grow when another mutation in the same gene occurs in a critical duct cell of the breast. Over 100 mutations can occur in this gene, so finding the mutations that are related to cancer is a complicated process. Further complicating the picture is evidence that the inherited mutations differ among families. It is thought that most families have their own unique mutation and that the mutation has arisen probably within the last few generations. The mutation is in DNA sub-units called nucleotides, and it causes the cell to shorten its translation of the gene's usual instructions for making a protein. Scientists do not yet know the complete function of the protein. Certain Jewish families (Ashkenazi Jews with roots in Eastern Europe, for example) are at high risk of breast cancer, and they have been found to share the same mutation in the BRCA 1 gene. However, almost 90% of United States Jews are Ashkenazi, and epidemiological studies give inconsistent results regarding whether Jewish women have a higher rate of breast cancer than do other women. Apparently, these are very complex issues.

Similar mutations shared by some families with shared ancestry have been found in Sweden, Iceland, and Scotland (King 1996). Studies are currently underway for African-American women who have multiple family members with breast cancer, since African-American women as a group have a higher incidence of breast cancer at younger ages than do other American women. The presence of gene mutations also seems to dramatically increase the risk of ovarian cancer and possibly endometrial (uterine) cancer as well. The gene mutations studied so far point toward an encoding error in DNA that affects repair proteins.

Evidence suggests that all cancers are probably the result of a gene-environment interaction, really. Either the gene inherited a problem or a problem in the gene was acquired later via hormones, pesticides, radiation, virus, or other mechanism we do not yet know.

The ability to screen for these genes is still in a very early stage of expertise. Presently, the test process is labor-intensive and expensive, and interpretation of the results is not completely accurate, resulting in an unknown rate of missed mutations. As of this writing, the screening is only available for the asking in a very few places in the United States; otherwise the screening is occurring in research protocols only. Genetic counseling and evaluation services are also available in very few places, notably the University of Pennsylvania Cancer Center. If you want more information on these studies or to see if you fit the criteria for being a participant in these studies, you can call the Cancer Information Service at 1-800-4-CANCER. Keep in mind that many of these studies will in fact not tell you whether your family has a gene that is being studied, because protocols have not yet been developed on how to advise women on what to do once they have this knowledge. Some doctors believe that because we cannot yet reliably prevent breast and pelvic cancers, it is unwise to test for the genes.

The same controversy exists regarding this screening as exists about the use of yearly or bi-yearly mammograms: both the genetic screen and regular mammography only "catch" a small percentage of cancers. Mammography fails to detect as much as 20% of all breast cancers and fails to detect as many as 40% in younger women because younger breast tissue is more dense and therefore harder to read on the mammogram X-ray. However, in women over 50 years of age, mammography reduces breast cancer deaths by about 39%.

All this means thousands of women are obtaining these procedures unnecessarily and thousands more actually have a cancer that is not found on the procedure. Yet, for that small percentage for whom the genetic screening or a mammogram was able to detect high risk or early cancer, these procedures are lifesaving. For some women, knowing the results of such tests may be empowering, but for others it can be overwhelming and anxiety-provoking. We have yet to find a satisfactory solution to this dilemma of who should get genetic and mammogram screening, for whom it is a wasteful use of medical resources or unnecessary exposure to radiation, and for whom it is too anxiety-producing and results in dangerous emotional paralysis.

A number of other genes have been found to be associated with breast cancer. These changes are not genetically inherited but probably occur during a woman's lifetime. Some of these genes are thought to be involved in the original occurrence of a breast cancer, while others are believed to be involved in tissue invasion and metastasis. These include genes named p53, AT, and GADD repair genes. Others being studied include RB suppresser gene, HER-2/neu oncogene, and genes that help regulate the cell's life cycle. No tests are yet developed to see who has these genes.

Also, problems have not yet been well addressed about insurance coverage for women in these families, because if a woman were to discover the presence of these genetic mutations in her family, she would possibly find it very difficult to obtain medical insurance (or life insurance and other insurances) because many insurance companies prefer to provide no coverage, or limited coverage, for what are called "pre-existing conditions," that is, a condition that was present before the women first purchased her insurance policy. Also, many insurance programs do not offer extensive coverage for "preventive" treatments, which would mean that these policies would not cover preventive mastectomy, preventive hysterectomy, or other preventive treatments that are yet to be discovered.

Breast Cancer

Breast cancer, and most other cancers, are described in terms of Stages. Staging serves several functions: It is a way to easily describe the extent and characteristics of the cancer; it is a factor in predicting survival or life expectancy of the woman with the cancer; and it is a guide by which treatments may be suggested. Treatments may include surgery, radiation, chemotherapy, other drug therapies, and so-called "alternative" therapies. Any one therapy or a combination of therapy modalities might be appropriate for a particular person.

A Stage O breast cancer is also called an "in situ" cancer; "in situ" is a Latin term indicating that the cancer cells are contained completely "within the site" where they originated and have not invaded surrounding tissue. In the in situ stage, a cancer does not have access to lymphatics or the

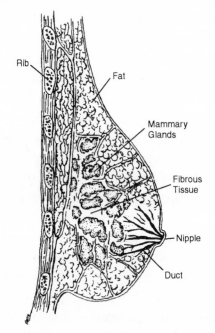

FIGURE 3. Side View of the Breast

blood vascular system; hence, it cannot spread to other parts of the body (i.e., it cannot metastasize). A Stage I breast cancer is one in which the cancer is no more than 2 centimeters in size and no cancer cells are found in any lymph nodes. Stage II indicates the cancer also is no bigger than 2 centimeters but has spread to the lymph nodes, or the cancer is larger than 2 centimeters but has not appeared in the lymph nodes. In Stage IIIA, the cancer tumor is larger than 5 centimeters and has spread to two or more of the lymph nodes, or the cancer is smaller than 5 centimeters and has spread to two or more of the lymph nodes. In Stage IIIB, the cancer in the breast has extended into other local structures, such as the chest wall or skin; it may or may not have involved lymph nodes in addition. In Stage IV the cancer has spread to a site distant from the breast, most commonly to the brain, bone, ovaries, adrenals, liver, or lungs. As you can see, each Stage indicates an incrementally more advanced disease, and as you might guess, the type and aggressiveness of treatment varies according to Stages.

In very advanced disease, treatments that take a toll on the body may be of little or no benefit or could possibly have an effect on function that compromises quality of life. Therefore, when a cancer is very widespread or the woman is very ill, she and her doctors may decide to discontinue treatments unless the treatments reduce pain or increase function. These may be important, even life-affirming choices to be made toward the end of life, and again, these are quite personal decisions.

For each of the Stages, many women have been medically followed for at least 5 years after their diagnosis, resulting in the following statistical survival rates. Studies show a fairly equivalent 5-year survival rate for early breast cancers (Stages 0, I, and II) whether the treatment was modified radical mastectomy or was partial mastectomy (lumpectomy) plus radiation therapy, yet this is a very personal choice for each woman. General overall 5-year survival rates for breast cancer are as follows: For Stage O, approximately 95% of women are still alive 5 years after diagnosis; for Stage I, about 80 to 85% of women remain alive after 5 years; for Stage II, the 5-year survival rate is approximately 65%; for Stage III it is 40%; and for Stage IV it is 10%.

These percentages may be both awful and relieving at the same time. The worst part, I think, is that you don't know which side of the percentage group you might be in. For example, if you have a Stage II cancer with a tumor size of 3 centimeters and just a few lymph nodes having cancer in them, you still don't know if you are in the 65% group who will survive at least 5 years or in the remaining group of 35% who will not. However, to help here a little bit, medical science is continuing to study additional factors besides Staging that may indicate both survival likelihood and how aggressive you may want your treatment to be. These factors include such measures as hormone receptor status (which measures how responsive the cancer cells are to estrogen and progesterone), the Grade of the tumor (which is a measure of how aggressively the tumor cells are dividing or how badly the DNA is out of whack), the type of cancer (lobular or ductal, for example), and other tests. The report that comes from the pathology laboratory where your tumor is studied microscopically will tell you this information. I highly recommend getting a copy of your pathology report and asking your doctors for an explanation of any terms you do not understand.

Some more recent studies that have followed women for more than 5 years are showing a slight increase in breast cancers in those breasts that were conserved (not completely removed) and were treated with radiation. This may mean that mastectomy is more likely to reduce the chances of a recurrence in the breasts themselves, which makes sense since most of the breast tissue is removed by the surgery, but note that it is not a recurrence in the breast that is lethal but a metastasis that is usually deadly. Therefore, knowing that a second cancer in the breast itself may not be deadly, many women may still choose a partial mastectomy or lumpectomy with radiation and plan to deal with a second breast cancer when and if it ever occurs, hoping to find it earlier rather than later. Others may feel that this risk is too great that even a small local cancer in the breast will have had a lot of time to throw out metastatic cells to other parts of the body by the time it is large enough to be seen or felt; these women may want to minimize this risk and would choose a mastectomy. However, note that even prophylactic mastectomy is not a guarantee that you will not develop a breast cancer, since a certain percentage of women will still have some breast tissue left after a mastectomy (and yes, even when it's done by a very skilled surgeon). Hence, the risk of breast cancer is greatly reduced by mastectomy but is not zero.

Other research indicates that younger women who have breast cancer are most likely as a group to choose breast conserving treatments; however younger women tend to have more high-grade tumors, more advanced disease upon detection, and to have poorer survival rates. It is not yet known if these poorer prognostic factors have any relationship to breast conserving treatment choices.

Elderly women with breast cancer are more likely to have their cancer discovered by their physician than by their own self-examination or by mammography. This speaks to the importance of regular physical exams for this age group. While older women more often choose mastectomy over lumpectomy when the outcome choices are equivalent, they are less likely to have their lymph nodes dissected and less likely to choose treatment with radiation.

Breast cancer that is discovered during pregnancy presents a difficult management problem, with conflicting issues relating to the treatment of the fetus and treatment of the cancer. Luckily, only about 3 cancers occur per 10,000 pregnancies. However, these cancers tend to be discovered in more advanced stages, when termination of the pregnancy is usually recommended due to the need for more aggressive chemotherapy and dual treatment with radiation, which could seriously or fatally harm the fetus. A woman certainly has the option to choose to carry the pregnancy to full term, but the trade-off is that she is likely to increase her own risk of an additional recurrence in the breast or additional spread of the cancer because of the delay in her treatment. This presents a most sad and serious choice for the woman herself and for her fetus.

The risk is unknown, but it presently appears that it is probably deleterious to mother or to child for a woman to become pregnant who has previously been treated for breast cancer. If her cancer was shown to be responsive to estrogen in the laboratory (this will be studied in the pathology laboratory after her biopsy or other surgery), it is theorized that high amounts of estrogen that are present throughout pregnancy would provide a hospitable condition for another cancer to take hold. Also, these women often have difficulty becoming pregnant at all, probably due to the after-effects of treatments and to age (few breast cancers occurring before the age of 35). This is another matter to talk over with your doctors before making a decision about whether or not to become pregnant.

Ovarian Cancer

This cancer appears in the reproductive organs that produce our monthly eggs that can be fertilized to have babies. *Ovum* is Latin for "egg." Ovarian cancer ranks second in incidence among gynecological cancers but ranks first in rate of death. (First place in incidence goes to endometrial [uterine] cancer.) Ovarian cancer is often called the "silent cancer"—80% of ovarian cancers are not discovered until they are in an advanced state with widespread metastases. Also, unlike breast cancer, there is no highly reliable early screening method. Substantial improvements have been made in recent years in being able to assign a useful stage to the extent of these cancers. This in turn has helped women receive more appropriate treatments, for example being treated with surgery only as therapy for Stage I ovarian cancers, with more aggressive treatments reserved for higher Stages.

One woman out of every 55 (a little less than 2%) will develop ovarian cancer in her lifetime. Cancer of the ovary produces few symptoms, so, sadly, most women do not find they have this cancer until it has spread enough to create pressure on nearby abdominal organs, and at that point the chance of living for five years after diagnosis is between 20% and 25%. For those women who do discover ovarian cancer very early, the survival rates are similar to those of early stage breast cancer, namely an 85% to 90% chance of surviving for 5 years or more after diagnosis. The overall 5-year survival rate for all Stages of ovarian cancer is 42%.

Many of the risk factors associated with ovarian cancer are similar to those of breast cancer; also, as with breast cancer, many women with ovarian cancer do not fit the high risk profile. Having other family members with ovarian or breast cancer does appear to increase a woman's risk of ovarian cancer, and to this end the Gilda Radner Familial Ovarian Cancer Registry was formed. Women who have two or more close relatives with a history of ovarian cancer are encouraged to register with this program (1-800-OVARIAN), which will keep one informed of the very latest developments in familial ovarian cancer research plus recommendations for management.

Cervical Cancer

Cervical cancer appears in the tissue of the cervix, the narrow lower end of the uterus that also forms the back or upper end of the vagina. *Cervix* is Latin for "neck." The use of surgical treatment alone for cervical cancer has increased in the 1990s from 26% to 33%. This is probably due to increased use of extended hysterectomy. On the other hand, the use of radiation therapy for cervical cancer has decreased over the past decade from 66% to 57%. In cervical cancer, the type of cancer cells make a difference in prognosis and treatment. Squamous cell carcinomas are associated with higher 5-year survival rates compared with adenocarcinomas,

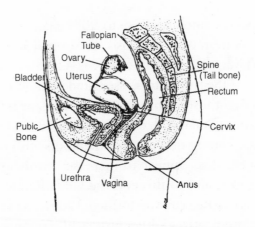

FIGURE 4. Side View of the Pelvic Organs

especially at the more advanced Stages of each of these types of cervical cancer. Because cervical cancers are often detected during obstetrical exams, treatments during pregnancy are common. Surgery is carried out with curative intent in approximately 70% of cases. A little over one third of pregnant cervical cancer patients are able to carry the pregnancy to fetal maturity, most requiring cesarean section for delivery. Detection of cervical cancer in later trimesters of pregnancy are associated with reduced survival rates compared with earlier trimesters.

Cervical cancer is usually discovered by a Pap smear test, which women are encouraged to get yearly as part of a general physical exam. The overall rate of cervical cancer has decreased steadily over the last several decades but has increased in recent years in women under 50 years of age. This is the one women's cancer that is strongly associated with a virus—human papillomavirus (HPV), the venereal wart virus. It is thought that this virus plays an integral role in the initiation of many cervical cancers but likely is not the only cause.

The Pap smear can detect precancerous lesions, called such things as dysplasia, low-grade and high-grade squamous intraepithelial lesions, and carcinoma in situ. It can also detect invasive cancer. Precancers are treated or followed carefully to minimize the risk of progression to an invasive cancer.

In very early stages of cervical cancer, such as precancers or microinvasive cancers, the treatment can be either simple surgery of the affected site, cryotherapy (the destruction of cells by extreme cold delivered to the cancerous area) or electrocoagulation (intense heat delivered to the cancerous area by electric current to destroy tissue). In more deeply invasive cervical cancer, more extensive surgery and possibly radiation and chemotherapy may be warranted. The 5-year survival rates are similar to those for breast cancer—from between 80% to 95% for Stage I cervical cancers, about 65% for Stage II, 38% for Stage III, and 11% for Stage IV. The overall 5-year survival rate for all stages of cervical cancers is 90%. But the mortality rate is more than twice as high for African-American women as for Caucasian women.

Cancer of the Vulva

Cancer of the vulva, the outer parts of the vaginal opening, has been uncommon among gynecological cancers, but unhappily it is on the increase, particularly among women under 40 years of age. Like most cancers, cancer of the vulva is most successfully treated if it is discovered early. If found only on the surface of the vulvar skin as a precancer or an in situ stage (Stage 0), treatment can be simple removal of the cancerous skin. If cancerous tissue is found also in the space between the vagina and rectum, surgical treatment often involves removing all vulval areas (vulvectomy), including labia and clitoris, and removal of nearby lymph nodes. For some of these patients, radiation only without surgery is considered. For more advanced stages of vulvar cancer, additional surgical removal of other affected areas can include bladder, anus, lower bowel, urethra, or vagina. In some instances, reconstruction can approximate normal function of bladder or bowel, but sometimes alternative openings must be created. Reconstruction of a clitoris does not appear to be possible, because the very dense contents of nerves in this organ that allow for orgasm cannot be replicated surgically. (Nerve tissue, which makes us capable of experiencing touch among other things, is notoriously poor at regenerating itself and cannot be grafted from elsewhere on the body). Additional radiation or chemotherapy are available for this cancer. Sexual activity, and sexual self-esteem, are often dramatically affected by this cancer.

Vaginal Cancer

Cancer of the vagina is another of the less common forms of gynecologic cancer. Young women whose mothers took the antimiscarriage drug DES (diethylstilbestrol) are at increased risk for vaginal cancer. DES use was discontinued in the U.S. in 1970. As with other gynecologic cancers, treatments range from surgical removal of the affected tissue in the early stages of the disease to extensive surgery with radiation and chemotherapy for more advanced stages. In the earlier stages, radiation can sometimes be delivered into the vagina instead of externally. Surgery usually removes the vagina in cases where the cancer is the squamous cell type, and it removes the vagina, cervix, uterus, ovaries, and fallopian tubes in cases where the cancer is an adenocarcinoma. Sometimes the vagina is reconstructed. Often lymph nodes are also removed from the pelvis. If the cancer has spread to the bladder or rectum, these organs are also removed and functionally reconstructed.

Gestational Trophoblastic Tumor

Another somewhat uncommon gynecologic condition is gestational trophoblastic tumor, which results from the tissues that are formed following pregnancy conception. If the trophoblastic proliferation is confined inside the uterus only, it is called hydatidiform mole and is usually treated with dilation and curettage (D & C) or surgical removal of the uterus. When the proliferation is found in the muscle of the uterus, it is called an invasive mole, or, depending on the aggressiveness, it is a choriocarcinoma. In this case, if there is no additional spread, hysterectomy and chemotherapy are usually recommended. In the most advanced stages, additional chemotherapy or radiation directed to affected distant sites is recommended.

Endometrial or Uterine Cancer

Endometrial cancer, the most common type of cancer of the uterus, is luckily often discovered in early stages and is often curable with surgical removal of the uterus (hysterectomy) and of the ovaries (oophorectomy) and fallopian tubes (salpingectomy). Additional radiation to the pelvic area may be recommended, particularly if cancer is found in the uterine myometrial muscle. Sometimes, endometrial cancer is discovered with a Pap smear test, but this happens more as a matter of chance than as a screening test for this type of cancer. (The Pap smear's primary goal is to detect squamous cell carcinoma of the cervix.) The 5-year survival rate for endometrial cancer is 83% overall, 94% if it is discovered at an early stage and 67% if diagnosed in a state with involvement only in the nearby regions rather than in distant organs.

THE TREATMENTS

The treatment options for breast cancers and gynecologic cancers can seem confusing at first, but again I advocate asking as many questions as many times as you need to in order to understand the treatment you choose, what it involves, and why.

Surgery

One of the most common treatments is, of course, surgery. There is little question that surgically cutting out the cancer cells is a highly useful treatment. Surgery is done to remove the cancerous tissue; nearby healthy-looking tissue is removed as well, for two reasons. First, the surgeon cannot see with the bare eye all cancer cells (this must be done with special tests and use of a microscope in a pathology laboratory), and second, if your own breast tissue or uterine tissue is "prone" to growing cancers, you may want the whole organ removed to reduce future risk of more cancer.

You then have a scar. Women have many divergent feelings about these scars. It can be a sign of amputation, or mutilation, or a loss, or a badge of courage, or a place of healing. Or its meaning may change from one thing to the next over the months or years. Here is a great, simple gift you can ask for from a friend who wants to be helpful but who seems not to know what to do for you: ask for a little bottle of vitamin E oil. Use the oil to rub on your scar daily (after the first couple days of initial healing). In the first months after surgery, rubbing in the vitamin E oil on the scar will help it become pliable, and the massaging action will help keep the skin from adhering tightly to the underlying tissues, as scars are prone to do if they aren't massaged regularly.

With the original cancer cells removed, they can no longer grow nor spread to other areas. However, a spreading process (metastasis) may have already begun that cannot be easily seen. Tiny cancer cells can be transported to other parts of the body through the bloodstream or through the

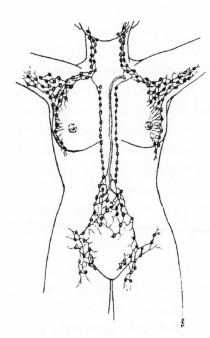

Some lymph nodes are near the surface of the body and can be easily felt, such as those in the neck and armpit. Others lie very deep in the body, such as those in the abdomen.

FIGURE 5. The Lymph System Network of Vessels and Lymph Nodes

lymph system, which is a network of small vessels that carry other fluids besides blood to and from many cells of the body. The lymph system has little "nodes" in some concentrated areas, particularly in the armpit, adjacent to major blood vessels, and in the groin. These nodes may do extra duty work to collect and contain bad cells like cancer cells. That is one reason some lymph nodes are removed at the time of surgery, either from your arm pit if you have breast cancer or from your groin if you have gynecologic cancer. If no cancer is found in the lymph nodes—even cancer small enough to only be detected under the microscope—it is less likely that the cancer has spread elsewhere than if cancer is found in many of the lymph nodes. This may be useful information to you in deciding how aggressive you want further treatments to be, or, it may be an unnecessary additional surgical procedure for you if you have already decided on your treatments. In either case, this is useful to discuss with doctors and other cancer survivors.

In years past, nearly all lymph nodes were removed, which often resulted in a painful and disabling swelling of the affected arms or legs which was called lymphedema (edema means swelling), caused by the inability of the destroyed lymph nodes in that area to carry fluids out of the tissue. Nowadays, only a sample of lymph nodes are removed, with the hope that the sample takes out enough of the nodes to know if there is cancer in them but leaves enough nodes to allow adequate lymph drainage in the limb. Still, because the lymph nodes are too small to be seen well, lymphedema can occur, so the surgeon cannot be precise about how many she or he is taking out; also, radiation tends to increase the likelihood of lymphedema to some degree.

One more note about lymphedema. It can also occur as the result of an infection, an insect bite, or circulation of blood constriction to the affected arm or leg. Plus, if such an infection does set in, it can be substantially dangerous, as your lymph system will be unable to handle a high load of infection in a way that it might have in the past and the resulting swelling could permanently destroy tissue by cutting off circulation. Thus, for the remainder of your days, it is wise to be extremely careful to avoid these possible sources of infection. You can do so by taking simple precautions, depending on whether the lymph nodes that were removed were in your armpits or groin: Wear gloves when gardening or handling sharp items, keep arms or legs covered from scratches or bacteria or insect bites, don't go bare foot, wash any cuts or scratches right away with copious amounts of iodine soap or "surgical scrub" (available at any pharmacy), have blood pressure taken or have blood drawn from other limbs, do not carry or place heavy items in a way that will constrict blood flow, and rest the affected limb in a position above the level of your heart on occasion to help it drain of fluids. If you're an avid outdoors woman like myself, take along antibiotics from your doctor and your iodine scrub if you're going to be out hiking or otherwise away from civilization for any length of time in case you sustain an injury in which an infection may begin.

Radiation

Radiation treatment is carried out by a radiologist physician with a team of technicians. Cell-damaging rays are aimed at the area where the cancer was removed and to nearby surrounding tissue to kill any remaining cancer cells. Usually this treatment is done on a daily basis (except weekends) for several weeks in a row. You are not radioactive yourself during this treatment, and you cannot hurt anyone by being near them. Sometimes an additional piece of radioactive material is placed under the skin for additional therapy, and during this time a short hospitalization is required because the radioactive pellet can emit radioactivity to others. Contrary to popular belief, radiation therapy to the pelvic area (for gynecologic cancers) and to the chest (for breast cancers) does not cause your hair to fall out; only hair that is directly exposed to the radiation can be damaged, so pubic hair can sometimes be affected in pelvic cancer treatment. But radiation to the pelvis can damage a woman's reproductive organs, making it difficult or impossible to have children later or interfering with menstrual cycles and hormone balances.

Radiation treatment makes most women very fatigued and often leaves some skin changes to the area that was radiated, such as a change in skin color or texture or sensitivity. Ironically, exposure to radiation is a *cause* of cancer, but medical experts are attempting to provide radiation treatment at low enough doses to not produce another cancer in you 20 years down the road yet enough radiation to kill the present cancer cells. This is not a perfect science yet. If you have asthma or other disorders that reduce your lung capacity, you may not be a candidate for radiation treatments after breast cancer because the radiation can sometimes further damage your lungs.

As with care of surgical scars, tender loving care of irradiated skin is a good idea. Ask your doctors about appropriate salves; also, you may want to consult a nutritionist or naturopathic expert for ideas on taking supplements or remedies to assist your tissue in repairing itself. As for the fatigue, listen to it! If you feel tired, it's because you need the rest. The body's activity in repairing damaged tissue is very energy depleting, and you may need and deserve substantially more rest than usual. Remember that cells repair themselves best when we're sleeping.

Chemotherapy

Chemotherapy is altogether different from radiation and is especially recommended if the cancer is likely to have spread beyond its original site in the body. This form of therapy can kill cancer cells anywhere in the body, whereas with radiation, only cells in the targeted body area are killed. Chemotherapy consists of strong drugs—poisons really— that are given directly into your bloodstream (although a few chemotherapy agents are given by mouth). Usually, you are given a combination of two or more chemotherapy drugs plus an agent or two to help the body recover—the mixture is called a "chemotherapy soup" or "cocktail."

These drugs have the capacity to kill certain kinds of cells, especially those that frequently replicate themselves. Such cells include cancer cells, but unfortunately, some normal cells are also vulnerable, like the cells that line your mouth and digestive tract, blood cells in the bone marrow, the cells that fight infections, and the cells that form your hair follicles. Not all chemotherapy drugs make your hair fall out and give you mouth sores and digestive trouble and seriously compromise your immune system, but many do. If you do lose the hair on your head, you are likely to lose hair elsewhere, too—like eyebrows and pubic hair—but not always. It's a difficult price to pay to help insure the destruction of more cancer cells and a decision that only each woman can make for herself.

Chemotherapy is usually not done on a daily basis like radiation is. Usually, a few weeks between doses is needed for the body to recover from the destruction of the "good" cells along with all the "bad" cells. Once a chemotherapy drug has been given for a full course (usually 4 to 12 times), it will usually not be effective against your cancer anymore. Any of your cancer cells that lived through that much chemotherapy have probably found a way to be resistant or mutate themselves, and if you were to need more chemotherapy in the future, other drugs will have to be used. This makes the choices harder when deciding whether to use more aggressive chemotherapy drugs the first time around—when you are hoping you won't ever need chemotherapy again—or to save the stronger ones in case they are needed later in your life.

Since ovaries have cells that replicate frequently, they are often damaged by chemotherapy and render a woman sterile in the process of killing cancer cells. This is especially important to women of childbearing age and to women who are concerned about estrogen production, since the ovaries produce most of the body's estrogen. There is current controversial theory that the death of the ovaries is one of the factors that contributes to reduced cancer recurrence in the future—precisely because of reduced estrogen levels—but this is not completely clear.

Additional Therapies

A treatment that has become more readily available (at least for breast cancer) is high dose chemotherapy plus bone marrow transplant. During this treatment, patients receive such strong dosages of chemotherapy that bone marrow is destroyed. Bone marrow is the source of the body's blood cells. Therefore, the bone marrow is removed before chemotherapy and returned afterward. This treatment does show some promise, but unfortunately not enough evidence yet exists to assure women that this much more drastic, painful, and dangerous treatment has any better promise of outcome benefit than do less aggressive therapies. The National Cancer Institute currently is sponsoring four studies to compare the outcomes of standard treatment against the outcomes of treatments after bone marrow transplant.

Many additional drugs and treatments are available, and lest you feel overwhelmed, it's nice to know that many of them can wait for a while to begin them, so you have time to think about them and see what really fits for you. The drug Tamoxifen is often recommended for breast cancer, for example. It may be of help especially for women who are already past menopause. The survival advantage gained from Tamoxifen is that it causes a notable reduction of cancer recurrence in the breast, but it is somewhat less effective in treatment of metastatic disease. As with all therapies, the pros and cons of this drug should be talked about with your doctors and other cancer survivors (especially cancer survivors who have a cancer similar to yours).

Additional hormone treatments, herbs, vitamins, dietary changes, heat therapies, acupuncture, other homeopathic, naturopathic, and Eastern medicine treatments, and other treatment not in the typical Western medicine armamentarium can be very useful collateral treatments that each woman may want to read about or ask about, as suits her nature. These treatments really can be helpful. Perhaps the best resource for this information is a book called *Breast Cancer: What You Should Know (But May Not Be Told) About Prevention, Diagnosis, and Treatment* by Austin and Hitchcock (1994).

SURVIVING THE DIAGNOSIS

Just surviving all the *waiting* times that are part and parcel of a cancer diagnosis is a feat unto itself. We wait for blood test results, for scans and X-rays to begin (hold your breath, now exhale) and then for the results, for biopsy appointments, for pathology reports, for confirmation of the frozen section diagnosis, for our phone calls to be returned, for second-opinion doctor appointments, oncologist appointments, radiologist appointments, plastic surgeon appointments, chemotherapy appointments and then pray for the clock to run fast so the treatments can be over, for diagnosis and treatment planning appointments, for the indicators of successfulness of treatment. We wait for the surgery to begin (counting backwards, 99, 98, 97 . . .), we wait for our memory to function properly again after anesthesia, we wait to be able to lift our arms over our heads

again, or walk energetically up a flight of stairs, we wait for
our hair to fall out in unimaginably big clumps, we wait for
the nausea to strike. (One patient told me that she got so
nauseated at every chemotherapy appointment that it became a reflex; months after her treatment, when she bumped
into her oncologist at an airport, she became instantly overwhelmed with the reflex nausea and vomited right there at
his feet!) Maybe worst of all, we wait for the feared rejection from loved ones to occur. And on some level, we wait
for our death.

We need more models and guidance for How To Be
Severely Tried. My patients describe bearing the waiting in
many and varied ways: holding on to a friend, meditating,
moving, walking, dancing, studying, doing crafts, reading,
rocking, gardening, showering, listening to music, making
music, playing card games, petting a cat, being "fully present,"
or the opposite—getting distracted. The waiting times are
indeed difficult times, but you can make them enriching
times as well.

To help survive the initial diagnosis, I recommend to
all my patients: Read your pathology report! It contains much
descriptive information that is useful to you for making treatment decisions: the diagnosis of type of cancer, whether it
is invasive or not, the tumor's size, the tumor's grade, the
likelihood that all of the cancer has been removed ("surgical margins"), lymph node status (i.e., was there cancer
found in the removed lymph nodes), estrogen and progesterone receptor status if applicable, the condition of surrounding tissue that was removed, and other measures of
how badly your cancer is acting that may have some bearing

on prognosis. Each of these factors can give you useful data about your own particular cancer. This information is more understandable than you might think, and can be very helpful in making your decisions about which treatments you choose. Your doctors can help you decipher this information and so can many of the good self-help books on women's cancers.

One common thing that you might want to use to distract you from your diagnosis is television, even though some people will be critical of such a use of your now-more-than-ever precious time. I recommend it because it's so banal that it disconnects your anxiety circuits briefly. Also, it can be psychologically soothing to see a show you've seen before, and the repetition and ability to predict the outcome of the story is psychologically comforting. Or, getting absorbed in a story you've never seen before can be just as beneficial. This is especially useful medicine during the first few days or weeks, when you feel "like an earthquake victim clawing your way out of the rubble, a Hiroshima survivor wandering dazed and confused in the ruins of what used to be your city" (Hooper 1994).

Naturally, I also recommend balancing distraction techniques with brief immersion times. Many women need some times of fully submerging themselves in the metaphorical sea of their cancer in order to stay aware and listen for inner wisdom to help guide decisions. Some of my patients plan their immersion times very carefully—taking themselves to a favorite beach or a favorite tree in a park, for instance. Some go alone, some take a journal to write in, some take a friend or their dog. You can light candles, wrap up in a favorite blanket, cradle a memento of a friend or relative who has had your same cancer, drink a special tea, whatever suits your time of allowing yourself to fully embrace the meaning of your cancer for you so far. You may find yourself weeping or wailing, pacing, storming, rocking, shouting, or sitting still in fright. These are times to let the scary or hurt or weary feelings rinse through you like a wave, so that the feelings may recede again to a quieter level in the background. This could probably bear doing over and over again many times—perhaps for the rest of your life, although the intensity of the waves will diminish with time.

Both distraction techniques and immersion times need a third category of activities to even everything out—rejuvenation times. During the initial months of coping with cancer and surviving its treatments, it is wise to make rejuvenation one of your top priorities. I encourage my patients to develop a list of activities and places that they have found to be rejuvenating over their lifetimes, so that they have many choices to pick from when they get blue and can't remember what to do for themselves. The list should provide self-suggestions for ways to spend time, people to spend time with, and places outdoors and indoors that give the individual woman a sense of lightness, being present in time (rather than thinking of past or future), refreshment of spirit or body, and a sense of being at home with oneself and with the world.

One of the things that the cancer pamphlets you will run across are always encouraging you to do is to discuss your feelings with your doctor—as if medical doctors were trained at handling complex emotions (Hooper 1994). They are not trained for this, although many make good effort to develop skill in this area. Several of my patients have mentioned that they found it helpful to think of their physicians as very highly trained technical wizards full of the utmost in scientific information and experts in medical treatment skills. But most are not trained to be "Dr. Welby" from the 1960s television show. Physicians (except psychiatrists) are not at all trained in concepts of emotional health, in how people make good decisions, coping mechanisms, reactions of loved ones, and the mind-body-spirit union. For this, I recommend a psychologist or other trained psychotherapist. Because of these differences in training, you might find it best to have a *team* of doctors, psychotherapists, and other health practitioners to guide you through your responses and needs about your cancer.

SURVIVING THE TREATMENTS

Susan Love, M.D., a breast cancer specialist and women's health expert, has called the current state of the art in cancer treatment "a program of slash, poison, and burn" (Love 1992). It can certainly feel like that at times. And it is indeed sad that cancer treatments are still so seemingly barbaric. Yet, they're all we've got at the moment. And each woman can contribute to some change in this sorry state of affairs if the idea appeals to her by getting involved in fund raising, legislative activities, or medical research. These steps can even be a very self-healing action at a later point in one's cancer recovery. Meanwhile, we're left with sorting through the after-effects and some continuing decisions about treatments as the date we first heard our cancer diagnosis creeps farther and farther behind us.

The drive to understand it will probably continue. Why did this happen? Our brains are programmed with a drive to find explanations. Randomness and unfairness are difficult for our brains to grasp, but they probably do exist. Thus, if your own explanations are useful to you, go ahead and use them: you may see your cancer as a stress you want to reduce, a lesson you want to learn, a meaning you want it to symbolize, a challenge, an adversity, a strength, a situation you want to change, a loss pure and simple.

And if a scientifically "unproven" treatment or an "alternative" treatment appeals to you, why not use it in addition to any other treatment choices you may have made? I believe the bottom line about "alternative" treatments is this: choose the treatments you have some belief in. If you don't believe at all in the efficacy of, say, acupuncture and believe you would find it an uncomfortable experience, forgo it. But if you are drawn to it (listen carefully for those subtle inner voices) or like what you've read about it or heard from friends about it, why not try it? Acupuncture, some vitamins and herbal formulas, as well as many other of these treatments are shown to be of efficacy for some people, but perhaps not for all. Give it your best feminine-intuition guess and go for it, if it interests you. "Can't hurt, might help," a patient of mine who has had breast cancer is fond of saying as she faithfully takes mouthfuls of vitamins and plant products that her own efforts at reading and research impressed her to try.

No matter how loathsome their experience with treatment is, most women find the demands of radiation or chemotherapy in some way reassuring—"At least I'm doing something to fight my cancer" is a comment I have heard from many of my patients. During treatments, a woman may have frequent—even daily—contact with a medical team, who become part of her support and guidance network in an allied fight against a deadly disease. An avalanche of emotion can hit once the therapy has ended. Ambivalence and confusion arise, due to mixtures of joy and fear that the treatments are stopped. When treatments stop, some women feel more vulnerable to a cancer beginning to grow again. Thus, many survivors feel a *need for closure*, such as a debriefing session with the treatment team to go over what she's been through and what to expect now. Often a client and I will do this together in my office. And it can be good to do this with friends and family as well.

Radiotherapy and chemotherapy can cause emotional distress through both their emotional and situational aspects, but they may also provide relief from distress by holding out the hope for cure. Studies show that the more treatments she goes through, the more distress a woman is likely to experience. It is the systemic treatment effects—the ones that affect the whole body, such as nausea, fatigue, weakness, or pain—that seem the most difficult to bear.

Because the uterus symbolizes womanhood itself to many women, the loss of this organ, or loss of ovaries or of menstrual periods, can present deep quandries about feminine identity. After hysterectomy or other loss of reproductive ability, a woman will not get fat and hairy and develop a male voice, as some people believe (although a small amount of weight gain is common). If the ovaries remain intact in a premenopausal woman, she will continue to have normal hormonal function from the ovaries, unless they were damaged by radiation or chemotherapy, but she will no longer have menstrual periods because her uterus is absent. The absence of her uterus is unlikely to interfere with her ability to reach sexual orgasm, since the sensitivity of the clitoris does not diminish after these procedures; however, the absence of uterine contractions during orgasm may be noticeable to some women. Sexual intercourse or insertion of fingers may feel different due to the changed length of the vagina and absence of the cervix; such changes call for new experimentation with sexually pleasing activities.

Some cancer surgeries do directly affect the clitoris or other outer areas of the genitalia (the vulvar area), and for these women, sexual activities may change more radically. Some of the more invasive gynecologic cancers require more extensive surgery that may remove portions or all of the bladder, rectum, vagina, or vulva. Plastic and reconstructive surgery can remake organs that will function similarly (with the exception of a clitoris, which cannot be reconstructed since the organ primarily consists of bundles of nerves).

This is a wonderful piece of medical science, that some of these organs can be rebuilt or redirected so that their function in the body can be maintained. Yet, many women experience the reconstructed organs or diversions as not her "own." She may wrestle with despairing thought over these changes, and considerable time may be needed for her to find a way for this to all make sense to her. While her surgeon might be quite pleased with the functional results of his or her reconstructive handiwork, and rightly so, the patient herself may experience it with a high degree of mourning and a lack of a sense of "ownership" or belongingness about these new body parts. So many of my patients have uttered at one time or another about reconstructed breasts, "They're fine, but they're not mine."

When all or part of the intestine is surgically removed, a new port is formed called an ostomy or stoma. Body wastes are eliminated through this stoma into a pouch that is strapped to the body. An ostomy made in the large intestine is called a colostomy; less often, an ostomy is made in the small intestine and this is called an ileostomy. Some survivors live with their ostomies permanently, and others eventually can have the stoma closed and the bowel reconnected to its original anal opening. Ostomies also can take a lot of time and work to adjust to. They can produce smells and embarrassing sounds, they require careful attention to cleanliness, and they have an especially strong impact on a woman's sense of attractiveness, body image, and body integrity. On the other hand, physically an ostomy does not necessarily impede activity. Once a woman has gotten used to its presence and its function, sexual activities, job duties, daily activities, even sports can all be carried out after ostomy surgery. One of my clients found that she felt better about her new constant companion—the ostomy bag—when she colored it with decorations.

Most all women will have a temporary urinary catheter in place for a few hours or days after gynecologic surgery, but it will be removed as soon as the kidneys and bladder are back to functioning normally. Some gynecologic cancers, however, involve the bladder to the extent that it cannot be reconstructed. These women may therefore have a permanent catheter and bag that is strapped to the leg for collecting the urine after it leaves the kidneys. The bladder is then prone to infections from bacteria making their way up the catheter tube, and this needs to be carefully monitored. As with ostomies, almost all previous activities can eventually be resumed, and the presence of the catheter requires time and courage and perhaps even humor to learn to live with gracefully. But not without a proper mourning period, first!

After radiation treatments, several problems or types of long-term damage are possible. Many women do not experience any of these effects, but those who do may need extra tending to, extra support, and extra time to sort out their ability to tackle these problems from their own best vantage point. One problem that can occur after radiation is perception difficulties and memory loss and diminished motor skills from radiation to the brain or central nervous system. Radiation to the head would usually only occur if metastases to the brain had been found. A more common post-radiation problem for breast cancer and gynecologic cancer survivors is pain and scarring. The pain can be recurring, intermittent, or chronic. Sometimes the pain can radiate down the affected arm or leg. For most women, the painfulness lessens with time, but this does not happen always. Chronic pain presents quite an additional management problem, and a woman who experiences this may also have to struggle with states of depression and difficulties with motivation until she can invent a way to live with some enthusiasm despite her pain. Pain medications may help, but their trade-off includes lethargy, cognitive sluggishness, and constipation.

Hypothyroidism and hyperthroidism can occur on occasion from radiation to the neck and chest. ("Hypo" means too little, "hyper" means too much.) These thyroid gland problems can cause noticeable fluctuations in energy levels, among other effects, but can usually be treated with replacement of proper amounts of hormones. Another, more common, effect of radiation delivered to the chest or neck areas is dry mouth. Also possible are reduced production of saliva, diminished sense of taste, difficulty chewing, trouble enunciating words, irritated gums, and sensitive teeth. Sometimes this can be permanent.

Radiation to the pelvic area can bring on bouts of diarrhea. If untreated, diarrhea can lead to dizziness, dehydration and kidney damage and severe metabolic problems, so do be sure you are watched closely if you have diarrhea. It can be a local reaction to the radiation itself or it can be from a virus that took opportunity in your body when your body was weakened. In the latter case, medicines should be prescribed. (A viral diarrhea can also result from chemotherapy treatments.)

Lymphedema (swelling because of poor drainage in the lymph system) can occur from a combination of the surgical lymph node removal and radiation to the breast or vulvar area. Lymphedema can be either painless or painful. It can also be disfiguring and it can impede walking or arm use. And, as mentioned earlier, it presents constant and permanent threat of infection from cuts, burns, and insect bites, which a patient should be careful to avoid. Lymphedema can occur during the radiation treatment or it can appear many years later, brought on by an infection. Furthermore, an untreated infection in a limb with lymphedema can occasionally be fatal. Lastly, vaginal stenosis can develop after radiation to the pelvis. Vaginal stenosis is a thinning of the vaginal walls that can cause the vagina to shrink or stick closed and scar. Vaginal dilators can be used to stretch the vagina and keep scar tissue from tightening after radiation. Keeping the area pliable with frequent (once or more per day) massage with massage oil or vitamin E oil, not too lightly, can prevent or reduce this and other scarring effects.

Chemotherapy, too, produces occasional long-range unwanted effects. Chemotherapy drugs are very potent, and unfortunately they can cause more damage than just killing cancer cells and making your mouth sore and your hair disappear. These long-term effects do not happen to everyone but are a brave reality for many women. One type of damage that can happen from chemotherapy is neuropathy (nerve damage). It is very disturbing and functionally debilitating, causing numbness and tingling and muscle weakness that can make you drop things a lot or cause you to fall unexpectedly. The effect is sometimes temporary. It usually does not appear until several months after chemotherapy treatment. In taking care of yourself, plan carefully to avoid potential injuries from burns and cuts, and check limbs daily for signs of infection that may go unnoticed due to numbness.

Constipation can be another complication of chemotherapy treatment. Mostly, it goes away after the chemotherapy treatments are complete. Also, some pain medications, antidepressants, and other medicines can cause constipation as well. High fiber in the diet and drinking the recommended 8 to 10 glasses of water per day will help. In cases where constipation becomes chronic, the patient should see her physician for appropriate treatment that doesn't include long-term use of enemas or laxatives.

Some chemotherapy agents cause long-term problems to otherwise healthy organs. Kidney damage, ringing in the ears, hearing loss, lung damage, and chronic congestive heart failure have all been seen in occasional instances after chemotherapy. A woman is at higher risk for these if she was in less good health prior to treatment. Paying close attention to your body and its signals may help you catch any of these problems early and thereby minimize potential further damage.

Finally, a more benign after-effect of chemotherapy for some women is a quirky desire for particular foods. The craved foods are often ones that are high in fat or sugar—that is, what we often call "soothing foods." Most patients feel that a little indulgence here is quite appropriate. Some find additional, truly soothing activities to make good alternates. Also, after chemotherapy, some women are left with an inability to eat some foods—usually these are foods that became associated with the chemotherapy or with nausea or vomiting. We human beings have a rather strong, involuntary mechanism left over from Stone Age days that tells us to avoid foods that made us sick (just in case the reason we got sick was because the food was poisonous). This mechanism was very useful in those days when humans foraged for food instead of eating from predictable garden produce as we do now, but the mechanism lives on neverthe-less. And it's not easily changeable. One of my patients made it her crusade to try to inform all newly diagnosed cancer patients she ran into about this phenomenon. She suggested that once it happens, it's too late, and the best approach is to have a "chemotherapy food plan," as she called it. Her food plan was to never eat anything you really liked, only things you didn't really care about for the next couple of days after a chemotherapy treatment. That way, it will only be those foods that you didn't like that you would have aver-sions to later.

Here is another one of the difficult dilemmas about cancer and its treatments. Even the most optimistic studies reveal that in postmenopausal women, there is scant evi-dence that chemotherapy improves life expectancy at all. In premenopausal women with breast cancer, chemotherapy saves 10% to 12% of those who would otherwise die (Hooper 1994), more for those with advanced cancers and less so for those with early cancer. This success rate is very, very important for those women who fall in that 10% to 12% category but is certainly no consolation to the other 88% to 90% who took chemotherapy but didn't need it. Plus, you would have to have a crystal ball to know for sure which of these two statistical categories you belong to—the group of women who would have survived just fine without chemo-therapy (so you would know ahead of time not to bother with it) or the group who would have died without it (so wow, are you glad you went through all that). These are no small decisions that women with cancer are faced with.

Having cancer often improves our ability to live with life's unknowns.

When the cancer is in an advanced stage, chemotherapy is not really considered to be curative for breast cancers and gynecological cancers (Krakoff 1996). Instead, chemotherapy can be seen as sometimes being able to induce remission and lengthen survival time for advanced breast cancers. For advanced ovarian and endometrial cancers, chemotherapy is seen as able to induce some response and provide some prolongation of survival. For advanced cervical cancer, response to chemotherapy is considered minor with no demonstrable prolongation of survival. Here again, we are left with the difficult task of trying to know ourselves well enough to use this self-knowledge to guide our treatment decisions.

We can become exhausted with the effort of steeling our bodies—of tensing our bodies—against real or imagined looks, comments, and criticisms that come after surgery or during treatments about our "new looks"—baldness, mouth sores, limping, fatigue, skin pallor, constricted movement, one-breasted or breastlessness. This becomes another one of those items that calls for us to find balance. We need times of letting down, of honestly being overcome with fear or ill health, of looking and acting as badly as we feel. And just as much, we need the regenerative balances of nurturing, relaxing, and soul-feeding types of activities. The women's cancer journey is nothing if it isn't all encompassing.

Clearly, there are pros and cons to nearly every possible choice or effect of a woman's cancer. Can I emphasize it enough that there is no right way to handle your cancer? Neither the treatment choices nor your emotional reactions nor the personal meanings of cancer have some right way to be expressed. Yet there well may be better ways *for you* to make your treatment choices, better ways *for you* to listen to and work with your own reactions and meanings. Finding these better ways is a matter of listening, with balance and integrity, to your own inner stirrings.

AFTER DIAGNOSIS AND TREATMENT: WHAT THEN?

Now the era of extended coping begins. The woman with cancer now begins to turn the page, leaving behind the acute, emergency-mode of coping needed during the first days or months of diagnosis and treatments and doctor appointments. Now the page turns to an ongoing, longer-range, "you mean this really wasn't all just a bad dream" redefinition mode. The patient starts to take on issues in a more headlong fashion. She begins to take inventory, to regroup, replenish, grieve, seek her needs, rethink her priorities, find new values, and accept fearfulness. She keeps a place in her mind or heart where she knows what it feels like to possess statistical odds about her life but to not know which category she is in—the "good" one (for example, the 90% who survive 5 years) or the "bad" one (that is, the other 10% who don't). She keeps in her mind or heart a probable knowledge of what it is she will die from and how she will die, if not when; and she wonders if she'd rather die by getting run over by a bus or would that actually make her feel cheated of the kind of death she has now become acquainted with.

She will become replete with feeling the good and the bad of having experienced all this—her fears and appreciations lists grow longer. This enriches her. She will keep working to forestall emotional paralysis and instead keep her ambition focused on initiative, on "being the renewed, invigorated author of 'whatever is left,' " as a patient of mine likes to say. It is time to redream her dreams. New dreams that fit new circumstances. *She cannot go back to the ways she was before her cancer. And she is not sure she wants to.*

CHANGE

Surviving cancer actually is a fairly new notion. A woman who survives a woman's cancer faces uncharted territory of living with a frightening, "chronic" disease. Her body may not (a) look, (b) feel, or (c) function as it used to. This means there is a lot of "new self" to get used to. "My new self" is a term I often hear recited by my cancer clients, with a wry tone that reads, "I wish I hadn't had to go through this, but I must admit I like who I am becoming as a result."

After surviving surgeries and therapies, other issues of survival emerge. It is during this time that survivors are more likely to encounter delayed stress reactions, fears of recurrence, fear of job loss, loss of loved one's support, and to begin to deal with issues such as loss of fertility, alterations in sexual functioning, different body capacities, and body image. She will likely reevaluate her life purpose, her career, and her relationships. Many cancer survivors need time to mourn their life before cancer, to grieve over the fact that after cancer, things are never quite the same. Having cancer changes a woman in many ways; some changes are visible, like scars or fatigue, and some are intangible, like her sense of meaning or purpose, her relationships, her outlook. I'll say it again, there is no "right" way to feel after cancer. Whatever *your* feelings are, they are windows to information about how to create your own renewal.

Most cancer patients find at least some positive, beneficial changes in their lives as the result of the cancer. Interviews with cancer patients have shown that most all of us describe several of these enhancements as a result of our encounter with cancer (Yalom 1980):

- A rearrangement of life's priorities; a trivializing of the trivial.
- A sense of liberation; being able to choose not to do things that we do not deem important to do.
- An enhanced sense of living in the immediate present, with an inspiration to do things now rather than postponing life until retirement or some other point in the future; an increased appreciation—even joy—for each day.
- A vivid appreciation of the elemental facts of life: the changing seasons, the wind, falling leaves, colors, and aromas.
- Deeper communication with loved ones, putting more effort into relationships, having more compassion for others, and being aware of others' feelings.

- Fewer interpersonal fears, less concern about rejection, greater willingness to take risks, and feeling more self-assured and inwardly stronger.

These are profound life enhancements indeed. As a psychologist, I particularly enjoy getting to hear about these things from my patients. I never, ever have to ask a patient if she can find anything positive about her cancer experience. Rather, these enhancements are always spontaneously and joyfully volunteered as they are encountered by each woman.

At some point in the months after diagnosis, each woman will begin to say how she notices colors so much more vividly now, or how she feels less self-conscious, more "centered" in herself, or more sensitive to others than she used to feel. Many women will mention how important their special friends and loved ones are, noting that the depth of connections between her and her dear ones has been "shaken up like salt in a salt shaker," as one client of mine put it; the grains of salt have been shaken and re-settled, bringing some dear ones closer than before while other friendships have faded because of the cancer. She may find that some friends simply are not able to remain close after a cancer crisis, and a distance begins to form between her and these friends. Other people who seemed but peripheral friends prior to the cancer may become so much more close and cherished after the diagnosis. These rearrangements in the depths of relationships, though sometimes painful, almost always seem real and right to the cancer survivor.

Somewhere in her reading or information-gathering about her cancer, she has probably become aware that once a woman has had either uterine, breast, ovarian, or colon cancer, her risk of developing one of these other cancers is raised significantly (Runowicz and Haupt 1995). Studies indicate that fear of recurrence of cancer is higher, more severe, and more disabling among breast cancer patients than for other types of cancer, probably because the 5-year survival rate has less meaning for this cancer and a recurrence may develop many years later (Holland & Rowland 1989). Also, having had a mastectomy versus breast conservation (lumpectomy) results in no differences in women's levels of fear of recurrence. Instead, what contributes most to fear of recurrence is the increased number of surgical procedures (Lasry and Margolese 1991).

But fears of recurrence are present for every woman with cancer. These fears encompass many domains. She fears death. She fears a painful death. She fears having to go through this all again, the next time with probably a less hopeful outlook. She fears for her loved ones. She fears for her shaky, new sense of integrity and for her still shaky new definitions of her own womanhood and femininity. The layers of fear are many. Fear becomes a new companion, eventually a companion to be befriended and embraced, perhaps one of those areas of "weakness" we all must admit to. But a weakness can still be lived out with wisdom and grace and self-nurturing.

Adjusting to a body change is one of the more arduous parts of surviving a woman's cancer. In our society, women are given to believe that our bodies, and especially our breasts and genital organs, largely determine our femininity; our value is determined by the presence of these organs and how well they function—and for how they look. When a woman loses a breast or breasts to cancer, or has abdominal scars, it threatens her femininity and her attractiveness; if her ovaries or uterus or other vulvar organs are taken away, she may feel robbed of her sense of womanhood also, or her mate may deem her so. Emotionally, this can be very traumatizing. Even temporary changes such as hair loss, a swollen arm or leg, or fatigue can erode a feeling of physical appeal (Runowicz and Haupt 1995). Because physical appeal is so overemphasized, its potential loss goes particularly deep. It will require a new stamina of self-definition for a woman to come around to eschewing the society's definition of her feminine features and to remake more realistic and personally accurate definitions for herself.

Sexuality can be central to our sense of ourselves and the way we express our femininity; sex can be closely tied to our sense of health and well-being. We each express our sexuality in different ways at various times in our lives. We may establish emotional closeness to others via sexuality and other forms of physical intimacy. Cancer can change our view of ourselves as sexual beings, can affect our ways of expressing our sexuality and other forms of physical closeness, and can affect how a partner or other important persons see us, sexually, intimately. Some of the cancer's effect on sexuality and physical intimacy may be temporary, some may be permanent. The organs that are affected by breast cancer and gynecological cancers are closely linked to sexual responsiveness, and, in many cultures, linked to our perception of what it means to be feminine, to be a woman, and to be attractive and sexually desirable. It may be helpful to remind ourselves that sexuality is a whole-body experience or better said, a whole-body-mind-spirit experience rather than just a genital experience. This reminds us that there is much we can do to redetermine a renewed sexuality.

Some patients or their partners are relieved to be reminded that cancer is not contagious. Some people may never have learned that cancer is not contagious, and others may unconsciously carry a belief that a person with cancer is contaminated in some way and should avoid touch, especially near the site of the cancer. Also, some people believe that externally delivered radiation makes a person radioactive. These are not true. However, implanted radiation devices are radioactive; and the patient will be in the hospital while the implant is in place and visitors will be limited to short encounters to reduce their exposure. Once the implant is removed, usually after just a few days, no more radiation can be released to others.

In the case of breast cancer, women respond in widely differing ways to any sexually related impact of their surgery or treatments. Many women find their breasts to be highly erotic areas of their bodies, particularly the nipples and the closely surrounding skin. On the other hand, some women do not find this to be at all true for them. Many changes in this status are possible after treatments. Surgical scars can be either painful or numb, and this will usually change some over time. Loss of an erogenous area will call for mourning and regrouping. A surgically reconstructed breast can also feel very different from one woman to the next. Nipple sensation will be absent if the nipple is reconstructed. If one breast is reconstructed and the other is surgically altered to make the pair more symmetrical, the second breast as well may have different tactile sensation than it did previously. Radiation treatment also can change the skin's response to touch, sexually and otherwise. Some women find the irradiated skin more tender and others find it less so. And these sensations can change over the course of months or years.

Whether to have her breasts reconstructed surgically is no easy question for some women, and I especially encourage ample thought before making these decisions. Actually, taking ample time to think about this is no easy task under the present day social (and medical) push to have breast reconstruction done at the same time as the mastectomy. I do not wish to discredit this simultaneous procedure—it is ideal for those women who really know that they want immediate reconstruction. Plus, it also saves a woman from undergoing additional anesthesia if she were to have the reconstructive surgery done at a later date, and I do think the number of times we undergo general anesthesia should be considered seriously, as anesthesia does take a toll on the body.

However, the danger of the push for immediate reconstruction is that it may not give a woman the time she deserves to really consider her own values, after peeling away the values of the culture or expectations of others. While many women may indeed choose reconstruction after careful consideration, I do hope for it to be an unhurried decision. Approximately half of women have their breasts reconstructed after mastectomy, either at the time of mastectomy or later, and half do not.

There are several different surgical methods and different products that are available for breast reconstruction, including using your own muscle tissue, which should be discussed in depth to help you determine a best choice for you.

Using your own muscle tissue eliminates the problem of your body rejecting a foreign material and similar dangers. Yet, to move a muscle from elsewhere in the body results in inevitable weakness and imbalance in the affected area. I have heard some surgeons remark that a woman can get a "free tummy tuck" along with a breast reconstruction by using abdominal muscles to form the new breast, but this kind of "tummy tuck" doesn't remove fat and may leave you unable to pick up your grandchildren to cuddle them because of the reduced abdominal muscles. Sometimes back muscles are used instead, again possibly resulting in compromised ability to lift or to haul the lawn mower out of the garage, for example. Each woman is different in her choices, and for many the tradeoffs are well worth it, perhaps particularly for women who are willing to spend the effort on reconditioning their bodies to compensate for the muscle changes.

The use of silicone for breast reconstruction is highly controversial. Convincing arguments are made on both sides: that silicone is virtually danger-free and that, on the other hand, it has a tendency to leak and cause severe, debilitating illness. If you're faced with this decision, my best recommendation is to do as much research as you can, trying not to rely on one-person wonder stories nor one-person horror stories either. The use of saline solution is less controversial and probably less dangerous than silicone, but some people feel that the resulting reconstructed breast does not have a very natural bounce or drape to it. Many plastic surgeons have pictures they can show you of reconstructed breasts so you can have a better idea of what to expect. Of course, they don't keep many pictures of really poor results, and that is where talking to other women is the method of choice.

Remember that reconstruction will not restore sensitivity of the breast. Women give extremely varied reports of their satisfaction with reconstruction, although most say that they are reasonably satisfied. It is a decision worth your loving consideration and worth taking the time to do a substantial amount of research into the satisfaction of patients who have had their reconstruction done by the same surgeon you have chosen.

Some women choose to live proudly with the scars of mastectomy. Others prefer to use a foam-filled prosthesis they can pin to an undergarment, or a silicone-filled prosthesis that fits in a breast cup. Others feel it is important to have reconstructive surgery to implant the shape of a breast. It is a personal decision that rests solely with the woman. And no decision should be considered too vain! Yet, any pressure to hide, disguise, or keep secret a mastectomy is rarely healthy. You may indeed choose to remain private about this aspect of your life—doing so out of integrity—but to do so out of embarrassment, shame, or fear would be less healthy. Better to confront the fear and build a road through it. While many women are very happy with their reconstructed breasts, other women feel as this woman does:

After my mastectomy in 1990, I got strong messages from those around me to choose a prosthesis, reconstructive surgery, or an implant as soon as possible. However, I have chosen to live without any of these measures; I live "one-sided."

I believe doing otherwise encourages women to view their breast cancer as a cosmetic event rather than a life-threatening disease. They may even forget the lesson of serious disease: our Earth time is limited; use it wisely.

I live one-sided as a statement of pride, and I'm reminded of the words of Audre Lorde in *The Cancer Journals* (Spinsters/Aunt Lute 1980): "Prosthesis offers the empty comfort of 'Nobody will know the difference.'" But it is that very difference that I wish to affirm, because I have lived it and survived it, and wish to share that strength with other women. If we are to translate the silence surrounding breast cancer into language and action, then the first step is that other women with mastectomies become visible to each other. Silence and invisibility go hand in hand with powerlessness. [Sue Holling, Letters, *Ms. Magazine*, VII:1]

In the pelvis, the vagina and labia can be reconstructed if a woman desires, but several organs cannot be reconstructed—the clitoris, uterus, and ovaries. Women who choose reconstruction report similar dynamics as do woman who choose breast reconstruction. Most report that the new constructions don't feel like their own body parts did, either in sensations or in sense of ownership ("This works, but it isn't like the real me."). The sensations after vaginal reconstruction are not fully predictable, and some women will experience much numbness while others will experience pain. Women who are more satisfied with vaginal reconstruction are those who enjoy intercourse for its own sake, without the complement of orgasm, and who are willing to carry out regular dilation procedures to keep the reconstructed vagina from developing more scarring, adhesions, and hardness. Also, some women choose reconstruction simply because they want to have a vagina—an important aspect of their femininity for some women—whether or not they "use" it much. As with many choices presented by a cancer diagnosis, there is no right or wrong choice, just a woman's own individual choice, and I advise talking to more than one plastic surgeon before making your choice.

After a hysterectomy for some pelvic cancers, whether or not the ovaries are removed, women usually experience reduced sensation of pressure against the cervix and the abdominal lining and the absence of contractions of the uterus during sexual activities. Thus, even if the external genitals, especially the clitoris, were unaffected by treatments, these changes in sensation can affect sexual response—sometimes a little, sometimes a lot. If ovaries are removed, the ovarian androgens (certain hormones) are greatly reduced, often lowering sexual response. Even if ovaries are not removed, this hormonal change can occur because the surgery to remove the uterus interferes with blood supply. After hysterectomy or oopherectomy (removing ovaries), vaginal lubrication lessens. This, too, affects the perception of sexual excitement. Less lubrication can be helped by using a lubrication cream for intercourse or for inserted fingers or objects, and will make these actions more comfortable and pleasant.

A shortened vagina or the presence of scar tissue in the pelvis can cause pain during sexual activities. Frequent gentle massage can help here, as can using objects to dilate the vagina gradually. In cases where more genital tissues are removed, sexual activities, desire, and responsiveness may be affected differently from woman to woman, and I encourage talking to health professionals and seeking out other women with similar surgeries and similar experiences to get the broadest range of information.

When my patients remind me of these changes, I often find myself wishing for some form of Post-Women's-Cancer Candid Sex Talk Group or some such thing to encourage women to be creative and exploratory in finding new ways to be sexually expressive. Many women do indeed listen well to their own renewed sexual voices after cancer, but it seems a shame to me that each woman has to reinvent herself entirely on her own, when there is possibly a great deal of information and encouragement to share.

Sexual partners will hopefully play a natural and involved role in sexual rediscoveries. Women who are single and wanting to date often find themselves thinking a lot about how and when to inform future partners of their individual, and perhaps uncommon, sexual ways. Women with partners also have a great deal to contemplate in figuring how to encourage their partners to be supportive without being pushy, to be loving without being overly solicitous, to show desire without seeming demanding, to wait out sometimes prolonged periods of lack of sexual desire. Often, these conversations bring couples closer than they have ever been before. Sadly, sometimes the opposite is the case.

It is also perfectly legitimate if a woman finds that her sexual desire has waned altogether. Some women, after a woman's cancer, simply feel no sense of sexual desire. If a woman in this state also feels robbed of that sexuality, I would encourage her to interpret those feelings as signals that she indeed does want to find ways to be sexual. If, on the other hand, her sensation of asexuality feels instead like a new way of being in the world, a sensation of freedom or arrival at a new place—perhaps with some mourning for her past sexuality, but again with no present regrets—I would encourage her to read these signals as a true, new, integrated asexuality that does indeed fit. As with so many of these postcancer changes, they may or may not alter themselves as time goes by.

Temporary changes in energy, sexual desire, and physical comfort with sexual activities can be the result of chemotherapy and radiation, feeling sick, being in pain, taking pain medications, the presence of ostomies or catheters or ports, quandries about attractiveness or femininity, or just plain struggling with fears. Usual ways of sexual expression may be suspended or modified for a time. It can be helpful if a partner is part of a discussion with health care providers about sexuality, especially about which activities should be suspended as well as resources for when and how to experiment with new forms of sexual expression. Talking over sexual question with trusted friends and, of course, therapists, is also a good idea.

In advanced illness, most people assume no sexual activity is possible. It is probably true that many people who are very ill feel a very reduced level of sexual interest, but not all. Individual differences should be discussed and honored.

Fertility can be affected after cancer either because of removal of reproductive organs or from the aftereffects of treatments. Often, but not always, radiation to the pelvic region and chemotherapy treatments will render the ovaries sterile. And some drug treatments used for longer term control of the cancer can reduce fertility. The loss of ability to have children affects women very differently, of course, and can be related to age, partnership status, the meaning of motherhood, and the personal meanings and symbols of the woman herself.

When a woman loses her ovaries to cancer, or receives chemotherapy, or receives radiation to her pelvis, or takes Tamoxifen, she may experience a painful dryness and shriveling of her genitals. Vaginal and anal areas can become dry, cracked, and tender. Lubrication is usually needed both to make sexual activity pleasant and for everyday comfort. Vaginal lubricants are available at drug stores and pharmacies as over-the-counter products like Astroglide®, Replens®, or K-Y Jelly®. For lubrication, nonpetroleum products are suggested if you need to take precautions against sexually transmitted diseases and your sexual partner uses condoms. Petroleum breaks down the material that condoms are made from. So, don't use Vaseline® for this (it's made from petroleum), and do read product labels.

For women who may not have used vaginal lubricants before, doing so may affect sexual spontaneity, at least initially. As a matter of fact, for many women, sexual expression changes quite a bit after cancer surgery because of physical changes, pain, fatigue, ill health, or changes in her internalized sense of attractiveness and desire. Some women, of course, do not experience such changes and some even find a revitalized sense of sexuality after a cancer diagnosis. After mastectomy, some women still enjoy being touched in the area of the healed scar, others do not. The same range is true after lumpectomy.

Long-term and late effects of the therapies used to treat cancers are coming more to the attention of medical personnel lately. Probably for the simple reason that more women are now living longer after their cancer diagnoses, the effects of medical therapy occurring several years—even as late as 20 years—after treatments is being seen more. For example, abnormalities in nerve tissue, called brachial plexus neuropathy, can occur years after radiotherapy for breast cancer; this can cause the pain of sensory damage or motor damage in the arm and hand. This incidence is on the decline, probably due to the use of lower-dose radiation treatments and due to discontinuing the practice of having the patient change positions during treatment in order to direct the radiation to other areas of the armpit or neck.

Chronic fatigue can also occur, either early during treatments or much later. The cause is unknown. Some believe it is brought about by the additional energy the body must expend repairing injured cells. Others believe that bone marrow suppression is responsible. The fatigue can be so profound that some women say they frequently feel like "I'd better lie down or I'll *fall* down." This can affect one's sense of self, identity, accomplishment. Probably the fatigue should be listened to; your body is giving you a clear signal that it needs rest. Learning to accept a reduced level of activity, however, means there is one more after-effect to be addressed. Most women dislike the sensation of very low energy and will be faced with quite a challenge to reinvent a good quality of life based on these new capacities.

For women who were premenopausal at the time of diagnosis, the instant menopause that can occur during treatment brings a new meaning to the term midlife crisis. Abruptly, in a few weeks' time, you are plunged, medically speaking, into deep middle age; you are postmenopausal. Gone are the biological cycles linked to the moon and the tides, the inevitable ebb and flow of estrogen and progesterone, "the rich female humours" (Hooper 1994). You're now in a hormonal milieu that is shockingly alien, made all the more so by the estrogen-blocking drugs such as Tamoxifen. Women's cancers, which have as-yet unknown relation to hormone levels, bestow all patients with questions about taking the common hormone replacement pills. Research on the possible bad effects or benign effects of taking hormones after menopause is very scarce for cancer patients. It is thought that hormone replacement should be avoided because some women's cancers, at least in the research laboratory, seem to grow better in the presence of some hormones, but there is extremely little evidence from outside the test tube to verify this. Therefore, the decision whether to take hormone replacement, as with so many other decisions, will require that each woman gather whatever information she can find, from health professionals and "sister survivors," and yet she will still be left with a very personal decision that will have to be based on her own knowledge and beliefs about her own body.

"Psychosocial variables," as we call them in the field of psychology, can affect a woman's sense of self, especially her sexual self, because of "artificial menopause," that is, the menopause that occurs after many chemotherapy treatments, radiation to the pelvic region, or treatment with Tamoxifen. Some of these variables (Kolodzie 1996) are:

1. Attitudes and Expectations: A woman's expectations of menopause have been found to affect her sexual functioning during and after menopause. For example, some women expect that menopause will bring a sense of sexual freedom from pregnancy, and these women often experience the enhanced sexual satisfaction that they expected. Alternatively, negative expectations, such as an anticipation of decreased sexual interest or pleasure due to menopause often results in the expected decline in sexual desire and satisfaction. The fact that a woman's expectations about menopause often come true is a call for more widespread and accurate information for woman about menopause and sexuality.

2. Emotional State: For women who have experienced a chronic state of anger or anxiety or depression, a decline in sexual functioning often occurs after menopause. These emotional states can have an

effect on level of sexual desire, enjoyment, and orgasm frequency. Related to emotional state is the quality of intimate relationships. Here again, the higher quality that a woman feels her intimate relationships to be, the more she will express satisfaction in her sexual interest and activities after menopause (whether the menopause is related to a cancer or not).

3. Physical Symptoms. After artificial menopause, many women experience vaginal symptoms such as dryness, a sense of tightness, or vaginal discharge or itching. These can affect her sexual self-esteem by making sexual activities uncomfortable. It is thus most important that women be provided with information about the care of their symptoms, about the use of lubricants, and about the many alternatives to intercourse that bring sexual satisfaction.

Most women do not learn about the consequences of having their lymph nodes tampered with until after the fact. Not being told the consequences before the procedure in itself can cause some turmoil and another layer of reactivity to cope with. For women who have had some or all lymph nodes removed surgically, every scratch and every cut becomes, as one client of mine says, a potential "ER Trauma." Every bug bite, every scratch, every kitchen cut, every razor cut, every burn and scrape, every walk through the brambles can (and perhaps should) find you examining your body for evidence of infection that may not be able to heal properly because of the lymph system's reduced ability to assist in defense.

We have become an army of women who develop an unnatural fear of razors, and whose weapon arsenals consist of a cache of antibiotic creams, iodine scrubs, and Band-Aids®. I keep these items ever at my side, in my travel bag, at my office, at home, in the barn, in my camping kit, in my car, unwilling to take the chance that *any* break in my skin could get too loaded with infection and result in permanent lymphedema or life-threatening infection. I keep even tiny wounds covered for days and days until the skin seems completely healed. (I wonder sometimes if I should buy stock in Band-Aids®or Curads®!) Since these little bandages have become nearly daily fashion wear for my fingers, friends often give me bandages with special designs, just for extra decor—glow in the dark bandages, star-covered bandages, and currently I wear Lion King® bandages because I'm fond of felines. Many of my cancer survivor patients make a nightly ritual of carefully examining their limbs, often with the help of their mate, to search for even a small dot or streak of red tissue that is the signal of an infection in the making. Vigilantly watching our limbs becomes a marker of our own burgeoning self-care.

The "anniversary phenomenon" happens to most women a year after their diagnosis, a herald of yet another change that cancer brings to our lives. It seems that as the calendar returns to the time of our diagnosis, something in us senses the familiar seasonal signals and remembers what we've been through. Women can experience this as either a sorrow and as a celebration. Or preferably, both. Often, the anniversary phenomenon occurs for years to come.

From anniversary phenomena to adjustment to body changes, to sexuality, to long-term treatment choices, the presence of changes in our lives becomes omni-present after a woman's cancer. Each of us was born with different propensities to enjoy change or to recoil from it. Either way, change may become a permanent com-panion, hopefully a companion that can be at least toler-ated and preferably embraced. The task of taking owner-ship of these changes becomes self-rejuvenating in the long run. In turn this can provide fuel for our journey of re-identification into our newly defined senses of femininity and womanhood.

How is it that a woman reconstructs her sense of self after her cancer? Most often it is an intangible process that begins with the initial reeling from the diagnosis and its per-sonal meaning to her. In this state, she is usually in a mode of psychological survival, and most inner resources are put to that purpose. Then a time that seems more like plodding rather than zestful living seems to take over for awhile. Dur-ing this state or phase, a woman can often operate in the world and even appear near normal in doing so, but she is mostly on "automatic pilot." It is as if our knowledge that we should eat or sleep or talk and so on carries us through these behaviors even though we do not feel fully involved in them. This numbness keeps us alive while we survey the disaster scene so we can begin to take stock of what will be needed to rebuild our lives.

Next often comes a time of extreme waves—waves of emotion, waves of exhaustion, waves of dependence often alternating with waves of fierce independence, waves of sor-row or fear or irritability or pain. During this time we are registering our losses and changes to their full degree. These sensations come in waves as a gift from our psyche, in that the psyche knows we need to be awash with the true depth of our experiences in order to move through them, but it also knows we shouldn't have to stand unremitting emotional pain, so the waves are allowed to recede awhile to provide a brief rest until the next wave washes in and over us. These are especially hard times, and because of the wave action, we may feel that we cannot tell if we are progressing or regressing. But progression does not mean the complete cessation of waves of difficulty; rather, progression means the slow lessening of the waves, both in intensity and in frequency, until they eventually become more backdrop than center stage.

This phase of waves eventually begins to overlap with the probable final phase of reconstruction of the self. Sooner or later, between the difficult waves, we begin to see moments of brightness, little appreciations, a returning ability to make choices that fit us. From these is born the belief that we can rebuild our own roadway for our travels. Also newly born, or reborn, is the sense of energy or know-how to build that road. The earlier phases have been the foundation required to now gather the necessary building materials and learn the skills of road-building for our lives. All the previous states we have been through since our diagnosis can now become the energy source to remake a life in which the unchangeable "givens" are incorporated with grace, and those things that we wish to choose and make for ourselves are available for the doing. Soon we can greet each day with enthusiasm and contribute to the well-lived lives of others and of ourselves.

3

The Search for Authenticity and the Role of Psychotherapy in Cancer Recovery

When a woman first learns that she has a cancer of the breast or of the pelvic organs, her faculties usually enter some kind of survival mode. The types of survival modes are numerous and may even be fairly unique. Some people survive by numbness, some by tears, some by paralysis, some by seeking information or support; some survive by denial, some by humor, some by spirituality, some by immersion in emotional states, and much more. Hopefully—for it is healthiest overall—a woman will find herself using many of these survival methods, each at one time or another, eventually finding which ones work best

133

for her under what conditions. The finest approach is the diverse approach—having many, many coping devices to choose from is the best state of affairs.

When she first arrives at my office, the newly diagnosed woman with cancer may be in any one of these states. In the waxing and waning of these survival states, she will probably begin to find meaningful threads of direction for herself. This is where I try to help the most. A significant part of psychotherapeutic help when working with women with cancer occurs by helping her expand the availability of diverse coping skills.

I took my training as a clinical psychologist, through which I learned skills of assessment and treatment of the many ailments and sufferings that can affect our minds, hearts, and behaviors. As a member of the allied health team, I have at hand many methods of helping and healing people in psychological pain or distress—methods that combine a medical diagnostic and treatment model with methods that can help people in ways that are behavioral, cognitive, mindful, emotional, heartfelt, and spiritual.

When a patient comes to me for help, my job is to sift through her experiences with her in order to develop a sort of "list" of both the causes and the effects of her discomforts. Once this "inventory" is made, the task switches to that of finding the methods of "cure" that will resonate as true for this particular woman. What is healing for one woman may not be so for another.

Therefore, simply telling a woman what the road is to her healing is rarely fruitful. Plus, humans don't learn very well by being told what to do. (If you're a parent, you've probably noticed this daily!) Rather, we learn best when the important factors are laid out within our view, where we can see for ourselves what it all means—especially what it means to us individually. For example, we learn more easily that $2+2=4$ if we are first taught how to count numbers (one, two, three, four, . . .), then shown four objects in pairs of two (one, two and one, two), and then shown how to count all of them (one, two, three, four) until we really comprehend that the two pairs brings the count to 4. If we are simply told to memorize that $2+2=4$, we will not comprehend why the answer is four, and we will be unable to add any other numbers.

As this example shows, my job becomes one of laying out the foundation work—as in teaching someone to count—or laying out the preliminary sketch, like an artist might do; perhaps I will paint or sculpt, in the psychological sense, what the patient is describing about her experience in such a way that she can see it in a new light, that she can see for herself that counting to two twice yields four, metaphorically. I then lead her, in a manner of speaking, further into the whole experiential window of this sculpture and ask her to open the window to make her vision even clearer and full of more detail, then to describe and immerse herself in the experience as she now sees it. This is the source of creative invention of her own method of healing. In doing this, she will come to believe her own perceptions to an appropriate degree and thereby be able to chart a course for living her life in a way that makes the best of her choices. I may explain new ways of coping to try. Or I may help her add additional perspectives, alternative behaviors, new details, insight, awareness of unseen motives, all of which will embellish the enrichment of her life, her experience, and her interactions with others.

I do not have all the right answers for my patients. What I have to give instead calls upon long-known methods of enabling a woman to find her own meaning, plan her own actions, see her own choices, seek the help she needs, and live with the degree of heartiness that she feels is true to herself, especially given the presence of cancer in her body—and especially given that cancer experience is occurring within the experience of being female, of being a woman. This is done with presence and with attention, by following her stories closely, by sometimes doing the steering for her and more often encouraging her to do her own steering by increasing her ability to evaluate her own choices, her abilities, and the outcomes of her thoughts and actions, by compassionately grasping what the presence of this cancer really means to her and her alone.

While much of my psychotherapeutic work with women with cancer is, in these ways I described, guiding, opening, experiential, and enhancing in nature, some of it is educational and informative as well. Thus, some therapy time is certainly spent discussing much of the information recited throughout this book. Women with women's cancers are often needing to ask, "How do I think about these things?" "What do I think about my 'quality of life'?" "What do I think is 'too invasive' a treatment for me? . . . " In addition to its educational quality, my psychotherapeutic approach touches on areas such as meaningfulness, roles, beliefs, self-esteem, and reevaluations, especially reevaluations of womanhood. The combination of providing education with providing self exploration leads to an enriched development of a woman's own "survival and recovery manual" within her own mind and heart, as one patient of mine called her therapy process.

The quintessence for me of this approach to psychotherapy rests in the establishment or enhancement of a woman's ongoing sense of the meaning of her life. The concept *meaning of life* invokes the composition of one's life that has the qualities of being alive and facile, a swaying gently within and among all one's traits and values and self-definitions. When a woman (or man, for that matter) can really tackle her own definition of the meaning of her life, I believe she will have the strongest foundation possible both to weather life's hardships and to amplify life's blessings. This approach to life is bound to be a guide that will make for few regrets and many riches, though every life must have both.

I mentioned in the first chapter of this book that I had asked a group of women to write their impressions and associations to the words *feminine* and *womanhood*. I also asked them to "free associate" to the term *meaning of life*. Their responses were as follows: *Meaning of life* means *ideology, creating, experiencing as much as possible, authenticity, self-exploration, questions, hopelessness, living with and through hurdles, grief and pain; coming to understanding, movement toward light/growth/unity/ love, development of self and community and world, to fully live, to find one's own meaning in life, "life is what you create it to be," to become, a journey, an individual discovery/invention, living as best you can day by day, to find the spark you came here with and put it out into the world, to live according to one's values, spirituality, to give back to community, expansion, leave something to improve the world, making a difference, to make the world a better place, to love, to help other people, participation, continuity, oneness, legacy, pleasure, finding the secret of joy,* and *happiness.* A few women left the card they were writing on blank, with a footnote that indicated, "This is not a failure to respond, it is my carefully considered response." The most common response refers to a theme of "authorship" of one's own life, and this is the very theme that my psychotherapeutic approach is based upon. *Authorship of one's own life* can also be actively pursued outside of psychotherapy, as many women do.

A large part of the psychotherapeutic work that facilitates patients taking full authorship of their lives is helping women with cancer discover what is replenishing to them individually. Together, the patient and I brainstorm all kinds of ideas, from tame to wild. Ideas flow, among them such things as baths in candlelight, special foods, favorite pillows, a worry stone, talismans and totems, play, change, discovery, nature, writing in a journal or diary, a reading group, a sewing group, taking advice from an animal, viewing art, inviolate time, comfort rituals, learning something new, saying affirmations, using scents, making a sanctuary, silence, droning sounds, enlivening sounds, play and laugh and be silly, growing things, touching things, rituals for loss, rituals for sadness, rituals for conjuring needed strengths. The possibilities are endless.

These activities lay the foundation for a more complete emergence through a woman's cancer experience—emergence into a renewed definition of womanhood, a renewed commitment to her personal meaning of life, and a reinvention of herself. An existential approach to psychotherapy treatments, which is the approach I find most germane to working with women with women's cancers, speaks primarily to personal meaningfulness and self-invention.

SELF-INVENTION

Psychotherapeutic styles come in many forms, and each therapist believes in the form she or he is using. I believe therapists gravitate toward a therapeutic style—a theory and basis for helping people—that fits their own view of the world. This is good, for it becomes awkward, and eventually ineffective, for a therapist to try to base her treatment style on beliefs that do not fit her individually. This is part of why each therapist adopts beliefs, styles, and techniques unique for her; and this is why each client may want to search awhile to find a therapist who is a good match in style and beliefs.

My psychotherapeutic style and training emphasizes existentialism. Existentialism has both a literary and a philosophical tradition, formulated by writers such as Kierkegaard, Sartre, and Heidegger, and formulated into psychotherapy by Victor Frankl, Rollo May, James Bugental, Emmy van Deurzen-Smith, Irvin Yalom, and theorists from closely related fields such as Interpersonal Analysis, Self Psychology, Gestalt Psychology, and Jungian Psychology. Existentialism holds that humans are wonderfully, totally free, and therefore painfully responsible for all our actions.

Also, existential thought postulates that humans completely create our own meaning of the world and its events; life therefore does not have a strict, known meaning that is the same for every person. Rather, each person's life energy can and should wisely be put to the search for personal meaning, within the community of human interdependence. It follows that cancer itself has a different meaning for each woman who has had it, for each woman who fears having it in the future, and for each of our friends and loved ones who encounter it through us.

While this therapeutic style goes hand-in-hand with a longer term therapeutic relationship and searching with a patient, it can also be fit into some aspects of the shorter term therapies that are commonly provided by some insurance companies now. Four to 6 psychotherapy sessions, the maximum provided by some insurance policies, is certainly not really therapy; but it comprises acute treatment or immediate problem solving and can have a place in existential methods, at least by lighting the spark to begin a quest for meaningfulness. But the process of broad discovery of meaningfulness is more of a journey than a destination. Thus to work this way in therapy can be a tack that occurs over many months and would be expected to continue after therapy for a lifetime, once the foundation is laid. And, of course, it need not be confined to psychotherapy at all.

Traditional psychology is often spare or entirely silent about deeper issues important to women: the archetypal, the intuitive, the sexual and cyclical, "the ages of women, a woman's way, a woman's knowing, her creative fire" (Estés 1992). Fortunately, the field of women's psychology has helped correct this problem and informs much of the methodology that I find curative in working with women with cancer. Because we are engaged in a day-by-day process of *self-invention*—not *discovery*, because what we search for perhaps may not exist until we find it or make it—both the past and the future are raw material, shaped and reshaped by each individual.

Also, possibly for women in particular, both the individual and the importance of relationships figure prominently in one's self-invention. "Composing a life" (Bateson 1990) involves a continual reimagining of the future and reinterpretation of the past to give meaning to the present—remembering best those events that prefigured what followed, forgetting those that proved to have no meaning within the narrative. Composing a life involves an openness to possibilities and the capacity to put them together in a way that is structurally sound.

To explore the creative potential of interrupted and conflicted lives, as cancer patients are called upon to do at least temporarily, is to exist as a bit of a feather in the wind, where energies are not narrowly focused or permanently pointed toward a single ambition but toward the nearby goal of simply surviving. These are not lives without commitment but rather lives in which commitments are continually refocused and redefined. We must invest time and passion in specific goals and yet at the same time acknowledge that these are mutable.

The existential position emphasizes and illuminates the conflict that flows from the individual's confrontations with the "givens" of existence—the inescapable, intrinsic properties of the human being's existence in the world. These "givens" are often noted as tensions between two opposing but equally important forces, both of which we need to find ways to understand and express in our lives in order to live most fully and authentically. One such "given" often discussed in existential writings is death—a core conflict between the awareness of the inevitability of death and the wish to continue to be. This also relates to our very common need to be special and the also-common desire for an ultimate rescuer. These two needs, to be special and to be rescued, are not infantile fantasies but actual yearnings within us; they are only problematic if we believe in them *literally* and therefore search them out as fairy tales that must come true for us to be happy. Rather, they are a *representation* of two important aspects of ourselves—the need to have our life choices come from within us (called "internal locus of control" in psychology) and the need to have a safe place to rest with the knowledge we will be taken care of while we are regrouping our strengths (called "external locus of control").

Another "given" commonly discussed in existential psychotherapy theory is freedom. Here, freedom means the absence of structure; the existential dynamic is the clash between our confrontation with groundlessness and our wish for solid footing and structure. In this view, the individual does not live in a structured universe that has an inherent design. Rather she is individually and entirely responsible for her own world, life design, choices, and actions. She will not be able to predict or control many of the things that happen to her, nor some of the tendencies she was born with, but all of these things can be taken on as her own challenge to make the best of them that she can. This concept implies the importance of *responsibility*, which refers to authorship, including actions and failure to act. I believe this is one reason why visualization techniques work so well and are often suggested as coping devices for cancer patients. Visualization is a method of developing images or visions of powerful symbolic actions, such as picturing your troubles being placed on a leaf floating down a stream until they are out of sight, or envisioning your favorite animal in miniature form being able to go within your body and seek out cancer cells and disable them for you. During visualization we assume a more active, responsible stance for our own treatments or illness.

Also, the notion of *willingness* is implied in thinking about the existential "given" of freedom. Willingness means the readiness to change and the disposition to accomplish change by our *actions*, not just in knowing, intending, promising, or dreaming. Willingness has a prerequisite: the ability to wish, wish deeply, emotionally, experientially. This is not the same as impulsivity—the undiscriminating, unthoughtful action to carry out a wish. Nor is it the same as compulsion—carrying out acts in accordance with inner demands that are *not* experienced as wishes. Our freedom as human beings is therefore both a wonderful, expansive ability to make a life of our choosing and a weighty responsibility to ourselves and to others.

Isolation is the third "given" that we existentialists are fond of writing about. The two sides of isolation refer to the tension between our awareness of our absolute isolation and our wish for contact and for protection, our wish to be part of the larger whole. No matter how close each of us comes to one another, there remains a final, unbridgeable gap—each of us enters existence alone and must depart it alone. No one else can ever fully understand our own unique experience. It requires inner strength, the sense of personal worth, and firm identity to face this anxiety and accomplish reasonably balanced forms of love and life. We remain separate-but-united creatures. On the one side is the anxiety of loneliness, isolation, absorption, which we all must experience from time to time; on the other is the joy of encounter, and communion with others. Both our dependence and our independence are forceful needs; if invited to integrate, they will accomplish a balance of interdependence.

Meaning—and meaninglessness—are the fourth "given" in existential theory. This denotes the dilemma of being a meaning-seeking creature who is thrown into a universe that has little known meaning. Living well incurs the question, "Can a meaning of one's own creation be sturdy enough to bear one's life?" (Yalom 1980). We seek coherence and a knowledge of our function: Why do we live? How shall we live? If we must die, what sense does anything make? Living well invites the ability to tolerate uncertainty and make something of it. The Eastern cultures of our planet Earth tend to follow philosophies that assume that there is indeed no "point" to life; instead, life is a mystery to be lived. Life requires no reason. Western cultures tend to seek meaning in good deeds or in expected rewards in an afterlife. Whether your thoughts follow more Eastern views or Western ones, a path must be laid that makes personal sense out of your

life. The search for meaning brings to focus the mixed blessings of our choices, which can result in either emptiness and
meaninglessness, or in the experiences of joy, beauty, and
ecstasy. Or preferably, both.

These dilemmas and tensions must be experienced before they can be transcended. It is the nature of human beings to be able to recognize and understand things best when
looked at through oppositions and contrasts. Thus, we will
understand the meaning of health through its contrast with
illness, of femininity through its contrast with masculinity,
of youth through its contrast with old age, of life itself
through contrast with death. This isn't morbid thinking, nor
pessimism, but a healthy route to discovery of the meaning
of our own lives. When one lives in a state of *forgetfulness of
being* (this is a common existential term), she lives in the
world of things, and immerses herself in the everyday tasks
and diversions of life. She is attending to the *way* things are.
She is unaware of her authorship of her own life and world.
In the other state, the state of *mindfulness of being,* she mar-
vels not only about the *way* things are but *that* they are. To
exist in this mode means to be continually aware of being.
She embraces her possibilities and limits, she faces absolute
freedom and nothingness, and is anxious in the face of them
(Yalom 1980), yet finds her way.

> . . . My idea of grace is fulfilling your talents com-
> pletely; my idea of sin is misusing that gift. The
> existential dread of not becoming completely what
> you can be is so strong that it can paralyze me. How

horrible to do the wrong thing, the thing that doesn't express your essence—and how horrible to fall short of your powers, or to discover that they might be more meager than their seemingly endless potential. [Hoffman 1989]

Even the simplest woman cannot remain simply "herself," purely female, if she is not to lose that most vital of all her qualities—her humanity. She cannot abdicate from the responsibility of consciousness, however rudimentary, and it is a responsibility which demands that she, no less than man, her brother, must never "cease from exploration" until she finds within her own being the sower of the seed, the creator of the light, as well as the passive earth; and all the time both man and woman are inevitably held in never ending tension between hubris ("I am the sun") and inertia ("I am the helpless victim"). . . . The point is that one must make incarnate in some form or other both the active sun and the passive earth of being. [Luke 1995]

In the existential view, all experience is interrelated and is organized by meaning. Meaning is not a cognitive or an intellectual term but encompasses thoughts–feelings–behaviors, (or mind–heart–body). Meaning is strongly conveyed by all the agents of culture (parents, siblings, media stories, relatives, peers, teachers) and is reorganized by each individual. Perhaps the most powerful principle of meaning is based on gender and is only secondarily intersected with other personal and cultural categories of meaningfulness such as race, ethnicity, sexual orientation, and class (Kaschak 1992).

> When either a man or a woman is saddled with a gender-based stereotype, his or her *humanness* suffers. . . . Neither the traditional man's role nor the traditional woman's role is desirable when one is trying to become a whole person with access to all of one's potential qualities. [Sullivan 1989, p. 15]

One real problem is an absence of passion and what seems a narrow range of accessing it and expressing it. We can lose touch with aliveness and joy, we fail to be *wholehearted* about our lives. We lose interest, excitement, appreciation. Not only do we suffer, but the community around us suffers as well because it loses the benefits of our energy, dedication, and spirit (Bepko and Krestan 1993).

My patients sometimes astonish me with their resilience. For example, one patient of mine had been active in psychotherapy for a long while, remaking a new sense of herself from the ashes of a very neglectful and abusive childhood. She was doing marvelously with herself: she had recently quit using too much alcohol, had enrolled in college to get her high school equivalency and reset her career direction, and had developed exciting new relational skills in her marriage when things began to crumble over a short span of time. Her brother was given a long sentence in jail, and my patient decided to raise his two young children for a while in addition to her own teenage children, which would interrupt her school plans. A sister-in-law was killed in a car accident and another sister-in-law was murdered in a store robbery. Her mother got breast cancer and then died suddenly of liver damage from a lifetime of alcohol abuse, which left no more opportunity for my client to reconcile some of her childhood experiences with her. She was in a motor vehicle accident while on her job as a school bus driver. Two teenage young men had careened around a corner head-on into her bus, killing one of the boys and causing multiple injuries to herself (there were no children on the bus at the time).

In the midst of all this, her doctor found she had a cervical cancer. Every aspect of her footing in life was under challenge. She put heroic effort into letting herself reel from the blows, and over time she was able to seek nurturing and support, grapple with the boy's death and the deaths of her relatives, face her own mortality, effectively manage several insurance systems—automobile, worker's compensation, and major medical insurance—faithfully exercise to regain lost function from her automobile injuries and from her cancer surgery, and remain involved and committed in her marriage. Despite her great hardships, she developed even better abilities to have faith in her own ways, to find meaning in tragedies, build strengths, and redefine her place in life, especially her femininity.

Her new view of her femininity included letting go of her need to rescue others' children (she'd done so more than once before), and she decided what was wise for her was to have her brother's children raised by other relatives, and she was able to return to school and to spare her teenage daughter the responsibility of too much child care of the young ones as well, another enhancement of her definition of femininity. And she navigated a renewed postcancer sexuality given the physical changes of her cervical cancer surgery. In addition, her husband became impressively supportive and involved, further enhancing their marriage. With time and effort and inner wisdom, the patient created new ground to walk on with a new existential sense of herself. She did find ways to come to peace about unfinished business in her childhood relationship with her mother. And she was able to live with the regret she felt that her mother perhaps had not been able to make something good out of her own cancer.

This is the existential sense: the inward vision that makes it possible for us to be continually aware of how well our outer experience matches our inner nature. The ideal of wholeness is a direction always to travel and never to attain. Too often we have chosen sides—spiritual versus sensual, behavior versus experience, self versus others, intellectual versus emotional, cautious versus spontaneous—rather than claiming the wholeness that is our potential.

For a woman with a woman's cancer, these subjects seem to arise for our contemplation as a matter of course. A dying person, of all people, is most drawn to the essential. And women who have had cancer have probably faced their deaths in deep and meaningful ways, and therefore have been drawn to seek what is most essential to them.

THE MAP OF THERAPY

Psychotherapy work requires much sensitivity, much ability to educate and to encourage personal research and searching, and much respect for individual differences. Each patient's course will be a little different from others', yet most of my therapeutic work with these patients does seem to follow a bearing that has these elements:

- Taking inventory of her own experience with her cancer
- Exploring the existential issues that have the most importance to her:
  - the meaning of death
  - freedom and responsibility, and the willingness to act
  - seeking a balanced interdependence
  - making meaningfulness from her life
- Adding to her repertoire of coping skills
- Reestablishing a style or ethic of relationships and caring
- Remaking her definitions of femininity and womanliness
- Discovery and reevaluation of areas of weakness and areas of strength
- Taking fuller authorship of her life, based on an integration of her real self and her ideal self.

The art of psychotherapy is one of acts of accompanying, evoking, and clarifying that give the patient a map to develop a sense of herself that is vital and authentic, one that embraces unchangeable "givens" and builds safeguards against ways of being that result in feelings of being derailed or depleted. We come best to understand the elements of our human experience through a process that organizes those elements, puts them together, assigns meaning to them, and prioritizes them (Mitchell 1993). Psychotherapy can facilitate this process greatly, although a person can certainly accomplish this on her own as well. Many women find, though, that these processes are enhanced when a guide, in the form of a therapist, is along for the journey. It's not that psychotherapists are necessarily wiser. It's that we are trained in a collection of knowledge about how the mind works and how experience is structured that are designed to be useful to the patient's own efforts to understand herself and thus to live with a greater sense of freedom, responsibility, and satisfaction in the world in which she finds herself.

The value of psychotherapists' knowledge is in the skills for making sense of a life, deepening relationships, and expanding and enriching the textures of experiences (Mitchell 1993). In applying this to gender, it is only recently that psychology has come to see that a healthy state of being is one that embraces both masculine and feminine traits, preferably traits that have been chosen after careful consideration rather than being subconsciously driven. At the same time that we try to develop a balanced sense of masculinity—femininity, it is clear that human beings have a need to establish a sense of gender, *either* masculine or feminine, as part of a stable identity. This is why an important part of the psychotherapeutic process for women with women's cancer (and perhaps for anyone) includes a reevaluation—and broadening—of the patient's definition of womanhood and femininity.

The dilemma often arises of how to answer patients' questions about my own cancer and my treatment choices. Patients tend to discern that my knowledge of the subject originates from more than just a place of academic or clinical interest. Of course, how much a psychotherapist shares of her own life is, in nearly all types of therapy, a matter for careful consideration. I make choices here that are based on therapeutic need, treatment plan, and assessment of boundaries for each patient. Primarily, I help the patient analyze her curiosity to know, to analyze how she thinks the information about my cancer will affect her. This is good practice for the patient on reading her own needs and motives, on building good ego strength, on being able to predict her own reactions, and, in particular, extending the boundary of being able to find her own path instead of following mine.

Psychotherapy patients can, of course, be profoundly affected by their therapist's experience with cancer. A patient who was in psychotherapy with me at the time of my second cancer experience wrote the following, noting how she interpreted what it was she heard from me and how she did and did not respond, which was worked through in later sessions:

Therapy Session #54

Flooded by my own thoughts
I enter your office ready to exfoliate
another layer of myself.

You are my safety
deposit box. A place where I learn delicately
to unfold my past lives in sections
like an ancient oriental
paper fan. Each fold uncovering colors
and textures, finally the whole scene
revealed. A place for inventing
my future lives. A place for both
to collide in a refolding.

I find my place on the couch
(it doesn't matter where
I start, I end up all over it).
Today your posture betrays you—
It's too late
you're sitting on the edge
unfolding before me—your life?
"I have bad news.
Six years ago they removed my breast.
The disease has returned.
They are removing my other breast."

My emotions lie still—
I am not the listener
in this "the listening cure."
Startled by my new role
I pick up a pad and pen.
Pressing on (I don't know if I'm breathing)
You reason out loud—

"Chemotherapy is out of the question.
I have no intention of voluntarily
poisoning myself with near-lethal doses."
I try to take notes.
Your mouth is still moving—
"My boyish figure about to be—is O.K.
with me."
Looking down at my pad—I know
there is no cure.

My innards try to escape
through my mouth and stick
in my throat.
My ribs want to burst my skin
one by one, buttons on a too
tight shirt.
I don't know how to fix you.
Mute and confused,
I say nothing.

You are living because I want you to.
You are living because I pay you.
You are living because you have to.
You are living because I need you to.
I need you to live so that I can finish—
move on. And, in three or four
years come back, a changeling,
a friend. Who can seek
your wisdom and laugh out loud with you.

Fifty minute sessions are where we live,
you and I. I want to talk to you
about you. Instead you settle back in your seat
and ask how my week was.
I fall back in step and describe
my latest hangnails.
You listen intently—
forever the therapist. I want to stop,
ask questions. *I know* the questions.
But we have been following the same path
for so long that we have worn a trench
and I don't ask.
I want to talk to you about you.

> *Are you scared—are you mad?*
> *What happens to me if you die?*
> *What is your favorite flower?*
> *Where did you grow up?*
> *Is your family going to be with you?*
> *Who is your family?*
> *Who is your favorite author?*
> *Who will take care of your animals?*
> *What is your favorite color?*
> *Who is taking care of you after surgery?*

I don't mean to not ask
questions. But you sit in the *armchair*.

> *What does it mean to have no breasts?*
> *Where does the cancer go to feed?*

Does it invade other body parts?
Will you leave a dismembered, rejected
lethal breast on an operating room floor?
Are you really O.K. to be breastless?

T.A. Godat

Printed with permission.

My patients respond in as many ways as there are patients. I love this diversity. Likewise, no two women respond in exactly the same ways to their cancer or their treatments. Some women experience searing, debilitating pain after surgery, while others are raising their arms above their heads to comb their hair on the next day after a mastectomy or are walking up stairs shortly after abdominal surgery. Some women are badly skinburned, profoundly fatigued, tender, coughy, or experience significant intestinal discomforts during radiation, while others breeze through it with barely a need for extra sleep. And chemotherapy is described by some as the most horrific and barbaric experience yet invented, while others bear it with only mild to moderate intermittent incapacitation. Dispel for yourself the notion that the minimal and easiest response that any woman has ever had to her treatments is the one you are supposed to have, too. There is nothing wrong with you if your body reacts in the stronger ranges of responses. It may just be the way you are built. Your life is for you to *experience*, not to pretend you don't.

I help women delve into a search for their apparent beliefs, their drives, their "old message tapes," in order to redecide them. This is a very important, and existential, process—a process of self-knowing, of learning to read and interpret her own inner experiences, what it is she perceives from the world around her, and what meaning she makes of those perceptions. This in turn becomes very consequential to the development of any new values, needs, directions, beliefs, and knowledge that will inform her cancer treatment choices.

The therapeutic work here is about new ways to be fully alive, not just accepting many cultures' emphases, such as the common emphasis on the body, for example. Instead, the client begins finding a truer voice, weaving a tight bond between her body and spirit, and redeciding her own values and the meanings of the organs and functions she may lose all or part of, temporarily or permanently.

Also, I can help women to know their own usual coping styles, and to add to them as well. When I first see these women in my office, more often than not they have taken up residence on one or the other extreme ends of a continuum—they are either in a debilitating, emotionally reactive or even paralyzed mode, or they are greatly *under*-reacting, too numb and distanced from themselves. These are common reactions in crisis. This coping mode must be acknowledged in a respectful manner before it will begin to dissipate—telling her she is over- or underreacting will in no way invoke her curiosity nor her ability to let the pendulum swing more toward middle ground, which are the eventual goals. Part of being "fully alive" includes temporary immersion in extremes. Once the crisis coping style is fully honored, it will almost always begin to soften in its strength, allowing room for adding less extreme coping devices.

One patient of mine had lived years beyond the original statistical predictions for her ovarian cancer but was beginning to experience repeated bouts of digestive difficulties, signaling a return of cancer that was interfering with her intestinal function. Each digestive crisis landed her back in the hospital, with a new treatment or procedure to alleviate her discomfort. And each of these crises landed her in a sequence of emotional reactivity that streamed from initial over-stoicism, to feeling utterly separated from her body and from her experience, to angry rantings at her caretakers, to what she called her "nuclear meltdown," to puddles of tears and inability to make decisions or carry out needed procedures.

After a few episodes, when this emotional pattern became apparent and predictable, she was able to work with it and modify it. She came to believe that she actually did need this sequence of reactions, but she found ways to express them that she felt much better about. Instead of stoicism, she came up with the idea of being "afraid-but-brave," she called it, which allowed the little bit of distancing that she needed at first, yet allowed acknowledgment of her fear. Instead of becoming utterly separated from her body and experience, she used distraction techniques such as listening to books on tape in her hospital room and keeping a dream journal and balanced this with asking loved ones for hand and foot massages so that she could feel good staying aware in her body. And instead of her "nuclear meltdowns," she invented a network of caring and helpful friends to tend her on a schedule, help her perform her medical procedures, and help talk over any decisions she needed to make. I was impressed with her ability to understand the meaning of her own behaviors and to find alternates that felt much more authentic to her.

Additionally, in my work with women with women's cancers, I emphasize relational aspects of living and healthy interdependence; these matters are shown over and over to be important to women. Also, the cancer is "happening" to loved ones too: husband, partner, children, lover, parents (for example, my dad cried over my cancer—a rarity, plus his mother had died also of breast cancer when he was only 14 years old—and my mom, who had had a cancerous tumor on her kidney several years prior said "Welcome"), other relatives, friends, sometimes co-workers and neighbors. Sometimes we don't even know who is affected by our cancer—others in the waiting rooms, store clerks who've heard about it, the nurse taking your blood pressure who herself has had cancer.

A woman's propensity to attend to relationships should, at some point, be turned to her own benefit in the form of social support. The importance of social support has been shown in recent research to be surprisingly strong. It is even possible that attending a regular support group or educational group may prolong life in cancer patients. Three kinds of support are often described: emotional support, informational support, and instrumental support, and you may want to make sure to incorporate all three, on your own or with the aid of psychotherapy:

- Emotional support refers to places and people where there is acceptance of emotional states and irrational states, acknowledgment that these states are mutable, and learning to read them as useful signals.

- Informational support means developing sources to get information, have your questions answered, and get help with decisions.
- Instrumental support refers to having practical needs met, such as being transported to appointments and receiving whatever assistance is desired with such things as preparing food or washing clothes or putting fresh sheets on your bed or help with bathing.

Psychotherapy, as you can see, is an art of calling on the client's own knowledge and learning style to build roadways to a more enriched self and a more enriched experience of the world and other people. It calls out her curiosity to broaden her views and believe in herself as the agent and author of a life only she can make meaning of.

4

Reclaiming a Postcancer Womanhood

In my capacity as psychotherapist, I do not—really, can-not—just hand a patient a road map to ideal healing and ideal living. Each person is so individualistic that such a map would never be able to cover each patient's unique de-velopment, unique perceptions and meanings, and unique needs. The patient's own psyche or spirit is the primary healer. My job is to potentiate that healing psyche by help-ing the patient gain self-awareness, self-understanding, com-petencies, and an increased ability to view her life from broader perspectives. My job also is to help open inner psy-chological doors that are essential to the process of living healthily. I help my patients learn to read their own signals better, incorporating difficulties in their lives along the way. Thus, I do not so much "cure" patients as provide hope and

attending that will activate a woman's own best inner curative responses. Psychotherapy may focus on the difficulties
of cancer experiences, but its deeper energy may come from
the impact of the patient talking about—and thus rejuvenating—her resources, her joys, her faith, her courage, her
solutions, her vision, and her new sense of authorship of
her life.

EMOTIONAL COPING: WOMAN'S HEART, WOMAN'S MIND

Humans seem to have an amazing resilience that no science or technology can yet approach: The body will enthu-
siastically repair. It will read its own need for coagulation,
tissue rebuilding, antibodies, sustenance—and dispense
these posthaste. So, too, is the psyche resilient, sending out
distress signals so we know there is something to attend to,
encouraging us to go searching for what's needed, and re-
vealing subtle signs of authenticity or a sense of going in the
right direction when we find or create answers and pathways that serve us well. Each patient is different in the methods and psychological bridges that open the necessary interior doors for her.

Thus therapists use many avenues to facilitate a patient's
growth, including exploration, practice, insight, behavioral
skills, cognitive restructuring, directed writings, hypnosis,
drama, role-playing, medicines, biofeedback, relaxation
techniques, readings, visualization and imagery, expressiveness, symbolism, communication skills, analysis, spiritual

exploration, and skills training, among others. Part of the art of therapy indeed is matching these modes to the individual patient's needs and character style.

Psychotherapy is an exquisite enterprise of listening to the patient's psyche, rather than directing it, and reading it back to her in ways that invite her to use her own inner information, along with external information, to chart her own course and develop her own wisdom. I will never be able to free her from pain. But I can help her invent ways for her suffering to become tolerable, meaningful, and even enriching, in addition to being inevitably agonizing and snarled.

Usually the whole family reacts to a cancer diagnosis, from children to mates to parents and grandparents, to siblings, aunts and uncles, cousins, blood relatives, step relatives, and chosen relatives. Likewise, networks of beloved friends are likely to have a series of reactions themselves. If these reactions are seen and talked about, a substantial net of support is likely to form as a result, both for the woman with cancer and for all those who care about her. Some reactions to look out for include the following: Shortly after receiving a diagnosis of cancer, most women experience a mix of many emotional and reactive states, usually including anxiety, fear, helplessness, anger, grief, envy, powerlessness, vulnerability, sadness, and aloneness (Kaye 1991). Early response to a crisis is often chaotic coping (Travis 1988). But this chaos, if allowed to take its course, eventually transforms into *strategies* for effective living. For most women, a gradual decline in these early emotional states occurs over the following couple of years as they are replaced with the new strategies.

As part of this process of decline in intense emotional states, many survivors report feeling a positive, existential change that is hard to describe. This positive change seems to encompass a clarity of priorities, with a reduced attention to what are now seen as trivialities and an increased emphasis on time spent with loved ones and an enhancement of priorities. Not all women experience this, but it is indeed one splendid outcome of a cancer diagnosis, one that shows the resilience of the human spirit. Other women simply report a sense of returning to "normal" over the months or years following their diagnosis. And a few others may find that they don't fare very well, feeling strong residual anxiety and vulnerability and lack of control. For these latter women, psychological intervention is called for and can almost always be substantially helpful.

Psychological researchers have identified some factors that are apparently quite helpful in helping cancer patients to cope, to reduce emotional distress, and even to thrive. One such factor, as I touched upon previously, is social support. Social support includes family closeness, understanding from spouse or partner, emotional support, social contacts, practical assistance with life tasks, and especially access to information. There are times, however, when social support can take forms that are not so good: for example, when friends, family, or peers dwell primarily on the negative side of the disease, then anxiety and lack of hope can increase. Also, families and friends who dismiss a cancer survivor's lingering fears and sadness, or ignore lingering emotional stuckness, can provoke anger or even more entrenched lack of hope or lack of action.

Some types of personal social support, support groups, and psychotherapy interventions, on the other hand, may be especially good. These include people and groups that provide an emotionally supportive context for expressing and addressing fears and anxieties and meaningfulness about the disease; groups or systems that offer information about the disease, its treatment options, and ranges of reactions, and groups or systems that teach, or help the woman create, the following:

1. Ways to behave (behavioral strategies) that help her balance her internal states with ways of regaining a self-directed position in her life, and
2. Ways to think (cognitive strategies) that do the same, providing training in relaxation techniques, imagery techniques, or enhancement of spiritual practices.

A goal of many methods of social support is developing realistic optimism. Optimism seems to provide a cushion of resilience to emotional distress. Realistic optimism doesn't mean denying the reality of the disease ("This isn't happening to me," or "I will go on completely as usual"). Actually, women who adopt this kind of denial approach for a length of time (it's okay briefly and intermittently) experience noticeably more distress in the long run than do women who accept their illness. Acceptance doesn't equal passive resignation or giving up; acceptance is an *active* process. Acceptance means discovering the ways the disease and its aftermath have actually affected her life, inside and out, and a willingness to enter this new life phase with real *engagement*.

Good *denial* is intermittent and serves to protect the emotional state of the patient from overwhelming waves of unacceptable or disabling emotional distress. It possibly helps build fibers of a bridge between the concept of self as healthy and the concept of self as having a disease. Denial is good if it gradually builds this bridge but does not go so far as to interfere with the ability to act on obtaining medical care or other forms of care.

Some degree of psychological *regression* is very common. That is, early on in the diagnosis and treatment planning events, a woman may find that she reverts to older, and therefore less effective, coping devices than any newer ones she may have developed in more recent years. This is an ordinary human phenomenon. When in acute distress, our reactions often feel preprogrammed to return to devices that were learned early in life that served a protective function for the psyche at that time. Often these earlier coping devices are more rigid and more narrow than more recently developed ones (of course, however, assuming we mature in our ways of coping over our lifetimes).

Also, earlier coping devices often have a shortsighted focus that can even contribute to less advantageous longer term outcomes. For example, overdependency may increase. Need for attention or to have others make decisions for her may increase. Preoccupation with herself or her (now difficult to perform) bodily functions may increase. Behaviors that elicited succor from parents in childhood may reappear. However, even though a woman may regress to these earlier forms of coping, they may be indeed real needs, and probably temporary. Also, most women will likely spring out of them spontaneously, recentering herself with newer more effective strategies, and probably she will even develop yet more mature strategies as she wends her way through the disease and treatment processes. If the regression becomes solidified, psychotherapy can help unlock it.

A patient of mine came to psychotherapy 2 months after his wife had been diagnosed with endometrial cancer; he was asking for help in "shaking her out of her emotionality." His wife, he said, cried a lot and seemed, in his mind, to act rather helpless. This is actually a common issue for mates and partners of women with cancer. My work with him was largely informative in nature, describing some common reactions to cancer that his wife may have been having, and telling him that two months wasn't a very long time to still be recovering. This work was very helpful to him.

But with a little time, he was able to study his own reactions to her reactions, and this is where the core psychological work resided. He uncovered his own profound fears that arose when his wife was scared or sad. In seeing this, he was then able to come to terms with the fact that he couldn't, and shouldn't, try to "fix her up quickly" by getting her to see only the good things still in her life. This was a useful piece of emotional work for the client himself, even though he thought he had come to therapy to work in his wife's emotions, not his! Further searching into his thoughts and feelings revealed another important aspect of his own recovery process: his profound sadness about his wife's lost womb as result of her cancer surgery. To him, having a uterus was a core aspect of her womanhood, even though they wanted no more children this late in life. It helped him greatly to discover this piece of his reactions, and gave him room to grieve his own losses. In doing so, he was able to engage more fully in his wife's recovery. I was then able to help him, and his wife as well, accomplish the task of fully understanding previous definitions and meaningful symbols of womanhood and femininity so that they could each evaluate and redevelop those definitions and symbols for the present and future.

Anxiety and *fear*, remember, are normal and necessary parts of psychological functioning, too. They signal us to be alert to potential dangers of all kinds, from physical dangers to psychological dangers, tangible to intangible dangers, some of which are difficult to consciously recognize, let alone to articulate. A women with cancer may have many such anxieties and of course they should be examined in order to give legitimacy to the dangers that she may want to actively address and to find methods of release or grieving for those that cannot be addressed or changed satisfactorily.

One client of mine I recall experienced a substantial amount of anxiety, enough that she began avoiding friends and missing doctor appointments. She felt she could not turn her mind off, which interfered with sleep at night and with concentration and memory during the day. She had breast cancer 12 years before, and had noticed abdominal symptoms over the past several months that turned out to be caused by an ovarian cancer. In our psychotherapy work, it emerged that her present anxiety was a stronger version of anxieties that she had experienced for a very long time. We explored how she had coped with this internal state for so many years, and she came to believe that "the heavy drinking days of my youth," she said, was a way to cover and escape the discomfort of her anxieties, and that since she'd quit drinking more than 20 years before, she coped by keeping somewhat frantically active, with little steady direction. Her children and grandchildren seemed to always be in some sort of difficulty, and she "flew around putting out fires and fixing things up for them." Also, she realized she had coped by exaggerating her role in the family as the everpresent but overly involved grandparent, her sole expression of her role as a woman, she said. All these were startling revelations, and she found them very useful. Further exploration and internal sorting led to beliefs that these roles and ways of living were much too narrow and that her anxiety had been a beacon signal all along, trying to bring to her attention the need to live less from stereotypes—and inward flight from herself—and more from deeper connection with her own values.

She set out on a mental and emotional journey to re-evaluate what was important to her, what was meaningful. With a great deal of journal writing, spiritual readings, and practice at using different ways of interacting with her extended family, she began to develop methods that would keep her on this path of inner authenticity. Despite a moderately bad prognosis for her cancer, she began to "grab my life by the horns" and become her own authentic life's author. Her womanhood, she decided, could be expressed not only with healthier activities with her grandchildren (activities that rescued them from trouble less often, and taught them skills for preventing the problems in the first place) but with more loving communication with her husband and in what she considered a feminine art form, knitting. Her anxiety still bothers her now and again, but she feels she now knows how to read it and she knows that returning her attention to living more fully and authentically will reduce the anxiety.

Grief is also a normal and healthy psychological process. It serves to prepare for and react to the experience of loss. Again, a woman with cancer may be facing many losses—some visible and others less so. Loss of health, loss of usual body function or a body part, loss of activities, loss of self-view, and threats of further loss are salient and legitimate privations. Grief often includes a preoccupation with what is lost, feelings of regret or self-recrimination, anger, a disruption of usual activities and viewpoints, sadness, physical symptoms like stomachaches, heartache, or headaches, a pining or searching for what is lost, and a wavering desire not to be reminded of the loss yet needing to be reminded so that the loss can be grasped.

These aspects of normal grief should be treated with support, legitimization, and understanding. They will usually come and go in waves, and these waves will gradually reduce in both frequency and in intensity over weeks or months. This gradually decreasing wave effect is the distinguishing feature between healthy grief and a prolonged depression. A deep depression will usually not be intermittent over time as grief is and will drastically affect self-esteem and motivation. This would be a marker for psychological interventions from a mental health professional.

Naming the loss and *describing the course* of grief can help the patient by helping her know what the trouble is (that it has a name) and by having a guide to know how most others respond and what she can expect herself. Generally, most people do not expect that losses will affect them for as long as they do. Unfortunately, our culture tends to praise people for getting over grief quickly ("She's back to work already and doing fine") or by refraining from showing grief ("She's so strong, she's hardly missed a beat. She's barely taken the time to cry over this."). These are not the healthy expressions of grief or fear. And if your cancer is one that will make you more and more ill over time, your grief will take on additional aspects, waves of possible despair alternated with acts of living well with your lessened capacities and coming to terms with long range debility and even your death.

Many women recognize a pattern to grief and recovery that is tied to the seasons. The first time "around the seasons" is often the hardest as we encounter each new holiday, weather change, birthday, and seasonal indicator from our new cancer survivor perspective. The second time around the seasons, as we encounter each of these markers again, our responses are more recognizable, and by the third time around, we often feel fairly well-settled into our new framework. This truth can run contrary to others' expectations that a few weeks or months is plenty of time for you to be encountering waves of grief or other discombobulating effects and their expectation that you should be "over it" by now. Guess what? You never get over it. That's right, never. And indeed you *shouldn't* ever get over it, not completely. It is an essential ingredient in your past in the makeup of who you will create yourself to be through your entire future.

I believe that the messages from others to hurry up your grief stems from their own discomfort with pain and suffering. It's wonderful that they want you to stop suffering as soon as possible. But if you care about your relationships with these well-meaning persons, you may want to "coach" them in how you want to be treated during a prolonged, ever-changing integration of what your cancer means to you. Let them know if you still want to talk about it. Or if you don't want to talk about it, perhaps, unless you yourself bring it up. Let them know if you want them to celebrate survival anniversaries with you (1 month, 1 year, 10 years, etc.) or not, or if you want them to still accompany you to doctor or treatment appointments long after you are able to drive or bus there yourself. And you can ask *them* what your cancer has come to mean to them every so often, as it may change for them as well as for you.

More than one patient of mine has found it important to develop specific rituals or ways of marking their survival anniversaries. One woman leaves her husband at home for a full week every year and travels to a small local resort that has mineral baths, massages, silent group meditations, and miles of contemplative walking trails in the Northwest Rain Forest. Another woman drives to the ocean with her husband and children, and they all make a special ritual of swimming together in the ocean to signify rinsing themselves clean of their losses. Another woman goes for a weekend retreat every year at a Catholic abbey. Yet another gathers her partner and several women friends who were her network of caretakers during her treatments and she cooks them an elaborate dinner. Some women make a special trip to their church on their anniversary day.

Many women and their families participate in the yearly "Race For The Cure," a walking and running event that occurs in many major cities sponsored by the Susan G. Komen Breast Cancer Foundation: this event is quite spectacular in some cities, drawing thousands of runners and walkers and often a few in wheel chairs—a sea of women and their supporters, with all the survivors of breast cancer donning a pink visor to denote their special status. And for my patients who are counting in months instead of years, often a small weekly or monthly celebration is still made as a sweet celebration of her life.

Having some choices available is core to many women's ability to cope with their cancer. Women who gather lots of information and from different sources usually feel better about how they grapple with their disease. This could mean having some choice in surgical options, such as partial versus complete mastectomy, removal of uterus or ovary only versus removal of all reproductive organs, retaining or removing the cervix, node dissection or no node dissection. Another area of choice is in how a woman may prepare for each chemotherapy or radiation treatment. Also, much choice should be available in areas of treatment beyond allopathic ones: vitamins and minerals, herbal, other plant or animal substances, dietary, homeopathic, naturopathic, acupuncture, hydrotherapy.

So, even if your first reaction is, "Give me a mastectomy, I want this cancerous thing off me," seek more information. You may well still make this same decision, but how much better you will feel about your decision if you consulted with a radiologist, for instance, to hear what the radiation treatments would be like even if you aren't going to get them; or speak with a plastic surgeon even if you don't think you're going to have reconstructive breast surgery or pelvic surgery.

Having control over these choices needs to be balanced with two things: the need for enough information to make good decisions and the need of the individual women to not be overwhelmed with too much information or decisions that are too difficult for her own personality style. Women tend to fare better who feel they had choices of their own. But listen also for a wise voice from within if it tells you to slow down, that it's time to stop gathering *more* information. There will always be more information to get, and the healthy trick is to find the point where you have gathered *enough* information for your own needs.

The Initial Impact and Loved Ones

When loved ones first hear about the cancer diagnosis, they may experience their own senses of shock, numbness, and disbelief. How and when to tell important other people about the diagnosis comes to the foreground for the patient and for loved ones; this should be discussed together so that both the needs of the new patient and her loved ones are balanced.

A noticeable number of my women cancer patients have a history of a parent's death where the parent was ill and at home for many months and the children were not allowed to talk about it with their peers, not allowed to bring school friends home, had to be quiet all the time at home, and were not told much about what was happening. Not only does this create some truncated ways of dealing with illness from their youth, but it presents current problems of management, both emotional and physical. These women benefit greatly from taking the time, in psychotherapy or not, to redetermine their own values about how the cancer should be mentioned to others. This process helps gain balance between privacy needs and need for care; it also helps gain balance between our own needs and the needs of others.

The diagnosis also may disorganize the usual ways of operating that occur within the family and within the support networks. Carrying out usual chores and routines is often difficult at first, but returning to a few comforting chores as soon as feasible tends to help a woman feel needed and important. Also, loved ones may be anxious and bewildered about what to do. Here again, discussion is important. Some people desire to be "protected"—from graphic details or complete information, for example—while others would be greatly disturbed, and disserved, by such withholding of information. The best thing to do is to ask each other what is wanted. Or experiment to see which you like better.

At this time, specific ideas ("May I bring you some soup?" "May I give you a foot rub?" "Shall I wash your hair for you?" "Would you like me to pray for you?") are usually more helpful than general ones ("Let me know if I can do anything for you"). Interventions that involve family and friends should be aimed at dispelling myths, such as the belief that it is bad for the patient to talk about her illness, or the belief that the patient is fragile and would be harmed by physical closeness. Also, priority should be placed on improving communication with direct requests and clear responses and facilitating both the patient's and the family members' expression of needs and feelings. Also, physical closeness should be discussed and encouraged if the patient so desires. One of my favorite memories of my second cancer experience was one of those "little things" that come to mean so much; as soon as we got home from the hospital after my mastectomy surgery, my partner plopped me in a warm, scented bathtub. We had to watch out for the bandages, but how indescribably good it felt to be washed by loving hands, to wipe away the smells and iodine stains of the hospital stay, and to begin a feeling of rinsing away the grief and shock. A perfect welcome home.

Children should always be given information and explanations they can understand and be given realistic reassurances, not false ones. Further, children should be encouraged to carry out both their usual age-related activities and to be involved in appropriate ways with care of the patient and running the home; in these matters, children of all ages may need a lot of guidance and two-way discussion. Young children especially are at a developmental stage where they tend to blame themselves or feel guilty for others' illness or death, and thus they should be helped to understand that any angry or scary thoughts they have are normal and are not a cause of their relative's illness.

Children will experience fears and disruptions caused by the illness of a loved one, especially if it's her or his mother. They should be told that thoughts cannot cause the cancer, and they may have to be told this again as they grow older and can understand this concept better. Common medical terms, rather than euphemisms, should be used with most children who are over preschool age; use and explain terms such as "cancer" and "mastectomy" and "hysterectomy." A child who "isn't ready" to hear information given to them will likely not absorb it and will need to be told again months or years later. For this reason, it is useful to bring up these topics occasionally over the years so the child can ask new questions appropriate to his or her age. As a matter of fact, I consider it quite critical that the subject of this cancer be brought up again every so often as the child grows.

Studies show that children's perceptions of the seriousness of their mother's (or other loved one's) cancer is quite accurate, despite how much or little they may have been told about it (Compas et al. 1996). The perception that they have little control over any aspects of the cancer's effects seems to constrain the types of coping options that are thus open to children. Therefore, one of the more helpful things we can do for children in these circumstances is to both encourage (and even teach) healthy expression-and-containment of emotions, plus give them little things they can have control over. For example, children benefit from such interventions appropriate to their age as choosing what to read to their mom, being in charge of a certain supply or a certain piece of the caretaking schedule, attending to phone calls or note cards, and so on.

Many adults are unsure whether children should be encouraged to attend a funeral or memorial service. The answer is quite simple—you will almost always do the right thing if you ask the child himself or herself. Explain who will be there, what will occur, the purpose of having a ritual of goodbye, and that she or he is warmly invited to attend but doesn't have to. Children too young to understand the explanation should probably be taken to the service unless they resist strongly. Years later it will likely be meaningful to know that they weren't left at home. If, for whatever reason, a child doesn't attend the memorial service, keeping pictures of it, or keeping a guest book, or a written memento may be very useful later for the child to review if she or he ever comes to regret not attending or has a delayed need to understand what happened.

A teenage daughter of a mother with a woman's cancer is in an especially precarious position and therefore requires special attention. Without enough consideration, the family often calls upon her to be "little mother" when her mother is incapacitated. It may indeed be useful for many teenage girls to be given a role to feel useful and engaged in their mother's illness, but this must be well-balanced with her need to stay active in her own age-related activities and to seek support from her peers or other adults in her life. Most particularly, knowing these cancers can run in families, at some time soon or far, she is likely to need considerable help with her own fears for her own health.

A college-age patient of mine is an example of these issues. An aunt had died of ovarian cancer recently, her mother had had breast cancer three years previously, and a cousin only a few years older than my patient had just been diagnosed with breast cancer. This patient came to realize that her method of coping with her mother's cancer had seemed good at the time but had left her feeling constricted and scared—and with a feeling of being one-step removed from her own experiences. She had been in high school at the time of her mother's cancer, in a very demanding academic program. Her father, I'm sure thinking this was wise, encouraged her to stay in the fast-paced program without a break, and he asked her also to add substantial household chores. For this patient, the balance was tipped too far in the direction of trying to go on as usual. In retrospect, it left her without the time she wanted to spend just sitting near her mother, or reading to her, and also left her too little time to talk about her experiences with peers and siblings. It was all these undigested experiences that was causing her to feel separated from herself.

As she came to realize these personal truths for herself, she decided that a good choice was for her to spend some extra time with her mother now, so she took a term off from college to create a special daughter–mother time and debrief both of their experiences with the cancer. This patient also had to find ways to grapple with the reality of so much cancer in her family and her own risk. She even considered preventive mastectomy—not an easy topic for a 20-year-old to contemplate. Emerging from her therapy on these matters, she decided to forgo the surgery but to study nutritional and lifestyle aspects of cancer prevention and carry these out to the best of her ability.

Engaging the Emotional Process

Everyone's feelings may become either very reactive or, on the other hand, very suppressed subsequent to the diagnosis. These feelings should be monitored, as they may be useful as an early coping device, but they can stymie emotional progress if they become more permanent. Some loved ones believe the new patient should be protected from displays of emotion, while others believe that she may want to see congruent expressions of such emotions; in regard to this matter, don't guess—ask her.

Further, a dark mood may not represent just an unhealthy state. It may be, instead, deep insight into one's existential condition at the moment. If a woman's response to her cancer goes awry, she is most likely to wind up with a full-blown depression or anxiety disorder. These conditions are very treatable by psychologists and psychiatrists as well as by social workers and counselors with specific training. Clinical depressions come in several flavors—called dysthymia, major depression, and bipolar disorders. These types indicate differences in frequency of depression bouts, depth of the depression, and whether manic episodes of overly high energy are present. Anxiety disorders also come in several flavors: generalized anxiety, phobias, post-traumatic stress disorder, panic attacks, and obsessive-compulsive disorder. These types represent differences in how anxiety manifests itself. With both the depressions and the anxieties, it is important for your clinical therapist to ascertain which type or types are present, because treatment differs among the types.

Clinical treatments for these disorders often consist of an appropriate form of psychotherapy, learning new skills, and sometimes taking medicines. Both depression and anxiety can interfere with thinking, interrupt sleep, affect appetite, and cause restlessness or fatigue. Because depression includes marked trouble with motivation and with decision-making, and because anxiety disorders interfere with concentration and function, it is especially important to diagnose and treat them early so the cancer patient can get back on her existential path. Other reactions that may signal the need for psychological intervention include adjustment reaction (a reaction to a stressor that is excessive enough to cause dysfunction), extreme bereavement, strong suicidal feelings, psychosis (a detachment from reality, usually with incoherence and hallucinations or delusions), and substance abuse.

Contrary to some assumptions, a review of the psychological literature reveals that most women cope well with their cancer and do not develop major psychological disorders. Only 25% of cancer patients seem to have significant depression or anxiety early after diagnosis (Schover 1991), and around 20% to 30% have significant distress of a prolonged nature (Atkinson 1994). While the cancer is highly distressing, women are remarkable in their ability for psychological and social adjustment. Even so, these percentages are disturbing given the sheer numbers of women who have, and will have, women's cancers.

Studies show that the patients who are most vulnerable to poor long-term emotional status are those with overly strong tendencies to suppress worries, withdraw, submit passively to recommendations and treatments, blame others for their plights, and remain indecisive. Vulnerability is also higher among patients who report relationship problems prior to cancer, who express regrets about the past, and who expect little social support. These patients also have more symptoms and a worse prognosis. Conversely, those with the least vulnerability are more hopeful, have fewer regrets and relationship problems, have fewer symptoms, expect lots of support, and have an active desire to live with problems that turn up (Weisman and Worden 1976–1977). Recognizing these vulnerable states is not reason for self-blame—rather this can be the first big step toward changing them for the better.

Some of the more effective coping strategies when you are feeling your worst are information seeking, mutuality with others, and resourcefulness in finding outlets—but only if these strategies lead to some resolution rather than becoming vehicles for endless questioning of decisions or alienating others or wallowing in unmovable emotions (Weisman and Worden 1976–1977). When left untreated, emotional distress can produce a substantial decline in quality of life and interfere with physical rehabilitation and needed social and expressive activities (Taylor 1990). If you think you are having more struggle with your cancer than seems natural, do consult a good clinical psychotherapist.

Re-dreaming Dreams and Framing Memories

Each person in the circles of family and loved ones, plus the patient herself, will eventually come to a place of new dreams that reflect a new, and possibly scary, reality. Dreams and memories may be either expanded or contracted, depending on the appropriate outlook for the cancer and upon the cancer patient's stage of life or view of herself in her life. Renewal of dreams is often a sign of healthy grief coming to completion; it represents the ability to take back the psychological energy that went into the grief and claim it instead as energy to reinvest in the newly defined future. Often, this includes a new relationship with time itself. Having "months to live" is the most common way that this information is delivered. After the initial shock, patients of mine who have heard these words reframe it to mean something more like, "Live well until you die."

Searching for Meaningfulness

Emotional and behavioral reorganization of family and friend networks builds the foundation for each person to find his or her own meaning in the cancer diagnosis. Discussions can be helpful to equalize tasks and consolidate resources. The diagnosis will come to be a meaningful event in the life of each person touched by its influence. Sharing these meanings as they grow and develop can be very enhancing for everyone involved, especially if each person is invited to create her or his own meaning. Here, as in so many areas, no one is more right than anyone else; it's the diversity of outlooks that is enriching.

Suppression

This is another frequently used emotional tactic. It refers to voluntarily excluding information, thought, or feelings from active awareness. This is often accomplished by focusing in another direction or by performing distracting activities. Since it is voluntary, the information or experience is available to the patient when she is ready. This is one of those strategies where a little may be good, and you need to be alert to what may be "too much of a good thing."

Displacement

This is the psychological term for coping by placing psychic energy from the area of intense worry to another area that is less conflicted or that feels less helpless. An example would be worrying more about your hemorrhoids than the cancer. Or about beauty. Or about others' reactions. This reaction is one not considered to be among the healthiest coping devices. If you notice yourself doing it, try chuckling endearingly at yourself and recognize it as a need to have some reprieve from your burdens. Then try a different coping device.

Overcompensation

One who attempts to deny the effects of the disease via coping is overcompensating. The denial is accomplished by efforts and behavior that would negate any disability or difference. Sometimes this can be good, as in the example of athletes who overcome a physical defect to become outstanding in their sport, or reconditioning yourself to run a marathon after pelvic surgery. Overcompensation isn't all bad but can be unhealthy when it turns into stoicism that endangers your health, like going back to work too soon after surgery. Use this coping device sparingly.

Mastery

Another intellectual coping technique that describes mastering a disease by learning as much about it as possible and acquiring lots of techniques required for care of the disease is mastery. This mode of coping is known to be an especially useful one. But even it could be taken to extremes if the intellectual aspects of your knowledge were to completely obscure the other aspects of the cancer, such as emotional responses and needs, spiritual needs, existential transformation. If you are like most humans, it will behoove you to put mastery high on your list of frequently used coping mechanisms.

Acceptance and Substitution

These are considered mature coping mechanisms. This means learning to accept (perhaps "embrace" is a more accurate term than "accept") the limitations of illness and then substitute and obtain pleasure from new activities. This is also seen as a healthy final stage of a grief process. Use these copers often.

Survivor Guilt

A phenomenon described by many people who remain alive through a tragedy where others do not is survivor guilt. It is a common feeling for people who live through a car wreck when others do not, or a flood, or a plane crash, for example. It is also common for women who have cancer and who are outliving other women with the same cancer. You might think it would make you glad to be continuing to survive your cancer, but sometimes the predominant feeling is guilt or sadness instead. It's a reversal of the "Why me?" syndrome, where we instead wonder "Why did I survive and not others?" It can leave us feeling overresponsible, or reluctant to face a friend with a worse prognosis from her cancer than we ourselves have. This is an especially illuminating phenomenon in cancer support groups, where some members of the group will die sooner than others. The survivors are left to remake their footing in a place of feeling luckier, or more responsible, or able to carry on a legacy from those already dead, or simply grappling with life's seeming unfairness.

One part of my own psychological healing was addressing the feeling of survivor guilt I had about the fact that I am living years beyond my cancers but my own grandmother did not. She had died of breast cancer at age 34, and her husband, (my grandfather) had also died of cancer, stomach cancer, a few years later. I never knew them, and my dad was still a teenager when he and his younger sister were left without parents. These cancers had ravaged his family, and I felt a sense of ancestral connection to this history I had known very little about. So as part of my reclamation and healing, I traveled across the country to meet my father's sister, whom I had never met before, to hear family stories from other relatives there, and, most importantly for me, learn about my grandmother. This became more useful than I knew at the time as I came to incorporate aspects of her that I had not realized were her legacy to me—her musical

ability, her love of cooking, her "green thumbs" in the garden, her psychological independence, and her dexterity with
home crafts. These were a form of deepened femininity for
me, my being able to credit my grandmother with unknow-
ingly passing these traits on to me and "doubling" for me
the effects of some similar traits that I take from my mother's
side of the family. Visiting my grandparents' grave site was
also an important spiritual ritual on my healing journey, allowing me to make better sense of my own meanings about
ancestry, legacy, and passing parts of ourselves onto others
who come after us.

The Effects of Trauma

When we encounter an adverse event, we are likely to
respond somewhere along a continuum that runs from *blunting* on one end to *monitoring* on the other end (Miller et al.
1996). A monitoring approach is one in which the patient
searches for information and amplifies especially the negative and threatening information, cognitively and emotionally; in a blunting approach, on the other hand, these cues
are strongly avoided. On the good side, a high degree of
monitoring can lead to obtaining broad useful information,
helping with treatment decisions, and a useful awareness of
the meaning of the disease to the particular women. On the
not-so-good side, high monitoring can result in chronic
worry, inability to turn off intrusive frightening thoughts, and
interference with effective problem solving. In a high degree
of blunting, the good results can be a protection from unen-
durable thoughts and emotions, but the down side can be a

frozen state of inexpression and, as with too much monitoring, an inability to make effective decisions. Like most polarities in human behavior, being at either extreme end of a continuum is less adaptive than being able to freely use aspects from both ends, and to do so moderately enough that we feel balanced and "in the middle" of the continuum a majority of the time.

The prevailing assumption in Western cultures is that it is good to be "in charge," as in "I've got to get control over myself," or "I should get control of my emotions." It's often considered shameful to admit that sometimes things can go very wrong, to confess that sometimes we have no control. But psychological trauma, such as cancer, overwhelm the ordinary systems of care that give people a sense of control, connection, and existential meaning. The signs of a trauma that has overwhelmed one's coping systems are:

1. Hyperarousal—after a traumatic experience, the human system of self-preservation seems to go onto permanent alert, as if the danger may return at any moment. Physiological arousal continues unabated. The person startles easily, reacts irritably to small provocation's, and sleeps poorly.

2. Intrusion—long after the danger is past, overly traumatized people relive the event as though it were continually recurring in the present. They cannot fully resume the normal course of their lives, for the trauma repeatedly interrupts. It arrests the course of normal development. The traumatic moment becomes encoded in an abnormal form of memory,

which breaks spontaneously into awareness and develops numerous, insignificant reminders and associations, making even formerly safe situations begin to feel unsafe.

3. Constriction—when a person is powerless and any form of resistance becomes futile, she may go into a state of surrender. The helpless person escapes from her situation not by action, since this option is not available to her, but, for example, by altering her state of consciousness by numbing or freezing.

4. Oscillation—the two contradictory responses of intrusion and constriction establish an oscillating rhythm—a hallmark characteristic of a posttraumatic stress. She finds herself caught between the two extremes of amnesia and reliving the trauma, lacking integration and balance.

5. Trauma calls into question basic human relationships. It shatters the construction of self that is formed and sustained in *relation to others*. It violates a faith in a natural or divine order, and it casts the woman into a state of existential crisis: of basic trust, of safety, of order, of meaning, of relationship to others, and of belongingness.

The ways of recovery from a sense of overtraumatization would include the following steps. First, it is essential to establish an atmosphere of safety and self-care, whether in a psychotherapy context or elsewhere. Next, a process of remembrance and mourning events, fears, losses, and wishes helps the psyche grasp the meaning of all that has occurred. Then a reconnection of interpersonal relationships and community is possible and should become the active focus (Herman 1992).

I've mentioned quite a list of coping devices and emotional reactions here. Psychologists thought at one time that some coping strategies—denial, avoidance, emotional expression, social support, problem solving, spirituality, humor, mastery, displacement, search for meaningfulness, and so forth—were more healthy than others. Further study shows that the issue is not really that simple. No one coping strategy is best—rather, the more strategies the better. This way, a woman can choose among several approaches whenever the need for coping arises. This not only feeds our legitimate need to have some control where we can but it allows us to experiment and eventually decide which strategies work better for us in which circumstances. This flexibility is a hallmark of mental health. The more proactive strategies—such as active problem solving, active information seeking, and active support seeking—seem to be the best strategies to use when there indeed is some realistic ability to control or change the stressor. The more emotion-focused coping strategies, such as emotional expression, avoidance, and the search for meaning, may be best to use when the stressful event is outside one's ability to control.

Again, when deep depressive symptoms or anxiety symptoms, including posttraumatic symptoms, persist beyond an expected normal reaction (roughly 6 to 12 weeks), psychological or psychiatric consultation should be sought. These symptoms would include persistent lassitude, anxiety, irritability, feelings of shame and worthlessness, crying spells, flashbacks, inability to "turn your mind off," anorexia, insomnia, decreased interest in activities, trouble concentrating or making decisions, withdrawal, and isolation. Watch for the presence of these signs—in yourself and in loved ones. If you see them continuing for several weeks approach with compassion, not criticism, and encourage proper professional treatment, whether it's for yourself or for another.

IT'S YOUR CANCER, IT'S YOUR LIFE

Research findings indicate that the more actively the patient participates in medical decisions and their implementation, the less devastating the illness and its treatment tends to become (Maddi 1990). Because this little fact has shown up time and time again in the literature in the field of health psychology, I'd suggest it be placed high on your priority list of ways to navigate your cancer experience. Even in areas where you feel you have no choice, try to find little choices. If chemotherapy treatments don't feel much like a choice anymore, try consciously choosing what to wear to the treatments, or what day to have the treatments, who to take with you, what music to listen to during treatments, what activity to do in the few hours before the nausea takes over, and so on.

A patient of mine described finding little choices for herself when she was confined to bed on a daily basis to place her arm in a compression pump to relieve her lymphedema symptoms; she chose inspiring passages for her family to read to her, she sewed decorations onto her arm covering, she called friends on the telephone while on the pump, she purchased special bed sheets to make the bedtime more esthetically pleasant, she watched comedy videos so she could laugh a lot while on the pump, and as a personal symbol to herself, she had a beautiful tattoo made on the arm that did not have lymphedema, a purple iris fashioned after the paintings of Georgia O'Keefe.

"Quality of life" is a concept frequently discussed in present days, but it is only a recent notion in medicine. Further, it has no agreed-upon definition. Patients' own rating of their quality of life seem to differ a lot from their physicians' ratings, patients referring more to a sense of worth or meaning or belonging and physicians referring more often to functional abilities. Some known factors that result in reports of poorer quality of life from both patients and their physicians do include unpleasant and debilitative treatments, problem treatment side effects, and functional impairment (Taylor 1990). Because these are factors that a woman does not have much control over, priority can be placed again on the little choices involved in these treatment effects to help enhance quality of life. Extra doses of self-care, nurturance, and contact with caring others will also lessen the burden.

The goal of maximizing your quality of life does not rely just on taking control and blind "positive thinking" but on something more like "realistic positive thinking." Again, the concept of balance appears, and it's a balance that each woman must find for herself and keep finding over her lifetime, because we are dynamic, changing beings, not stagnant unchangeable ones. This balance requires knowledgeable choices about what is worth fighting for and what is not, which can only be learned by our willingness to try and our willingness to be mistaken and to try again. And it makes room for a great deal of crying and sadness and terror, the dark side of our experience, so that we may also experience the light side—feelings of joy and laughter and passionate engagement in living. In these ways, hope becomes a vibrant reality. These experiences result in a sense of "living better," of having a better quality of life.

Quality of life can also be contributed to in many lifestyle ways. Many women, for example, report that physical workouts (even very short and slow ones) enhance their sense of confidence and of esteem, including their capacity to be sexually aroused. Exercise encompasses mastery of the physical and reintegration of a fragmented body (Kaschak 1992). To whatever degree you are able, physical movement of any kind should be a high priority. Moving, whether gently or vigorously, keeps our physical and psychological juices flowing smoothly and freely. I find it noteworthy that when I have asked women to name a time or two in their life when they felt their very best, the majority name a time when they were actively immersed in an activity that involved using their physical body and usually involved being outdoors. Further, research indicates that women who exercise moderately about 3 times per week have a cancer occurrence rate that is 40% less than for women who do not exercise. Because exercise is known to affect the balance of hormones, this is thought to be the reason for its protective effect, although the exact reasons are not yet known.

Laughter is another important ingredient in optimizing your quality of life. Not only does it feel really good to laugh (except perhaps when you are in a lot of pain), but laughter is thought to enhance the work of "natural killer cells." So stimulating your immune system is a great side effect to chortling your way through a comedy video, a favorite situation comedy, hearing or reading a funny story, watching children's antics or animal's antics, or otherwise playing in any way that appeals to you.

Your nutritional intake is also involved in an enhanced quality of life. You may be tired of hearing this, but in general, lean women feel less weighted down, have more energy, can stay more active and agile longer in their lives, and live longer. Eating what you need, rather than what you want, can be most rewarding, although I do not underestimate how difficult this can be. If it were easy to stay lean, everybody would be doing it! I think it is important to acknowledge how difficult it can be to eat what your body *needs*, rather than what it *wants*. But if it's important to you to be lean, try being respectful of any reluctance and remind yourself that you have done much harder, more fearful things than this.

Also, several nutritional elements have some research to support their usefulness in either cancer prevention or boosting the immune system. I'd recommend consulting a nutritionist or naturopathic physician for this, but it is worth your while to look into the benefits of a diet rich in antioxidant vitamins and minerals (particularly vitamin A, folic acid [a B Vitamin], vitamin C, vitamin E, beta carotene, and selenium). Obtaining these ingredients directly from plant food sources is probably more beneficial than taking them in pill form. There is also some recent research on the possible benefits of consuming fish oils and olive oil and eating hot peppers and tofu and other soybean products several times a week for prevention of women's cancers. It also appears best to avoid foods with high animal fat content (because of the concentration of hormones and pesticides that the animals were exposed to, as well as the role of dietary fat in unhealthy hormone fluctuations), foods that are smoked or charbroiled, foods that contain nitrite preservatives, foods that are highly refined instead of in their more roughage-abundant forms, and foods with high concentrations of pesticides or herbicides such as dried fruits that are not organically grown. There also is research being done on a possible link between women's cancers and consumption of alcohol; it is not known if organic wines would make a difference. Overall, the nutritional recommendation is to obtain most of your food from known, fresh plant sources.

Another ingredient in higher quality of life reported by patients is the sense of a peer group of other women with women's cancer who share the same religious preference or ethnicity or sexual orientation. You may want to seek out other single women with women's cancers, or other lesbians, or other Latinas, or other African-Americans or other Catholics or other Mormons, other DES daughters, and so on. Human beings have a strong psychological need for a sense of belonging, and peer groups such as these can provide additional buffers against the cancer's hardships.

A life of quality must include a well-modulated expression and use of emotional states. Our emotions are intended to provide "useful information." They are just one of our several methods of perception, like what we see with our eyes, hear with our ears, and touch with our skin. Ignoring feelings is the same as purposely closing your eyes all the time. However, using *only* your feelings or letting them overwhelm you is also not good. For example, imagine you see a lovely bowl of what you thought was fresh fruit. If you were using only one sense, your vision in this case, you might pick up an apple; if you ignored your sense of touch that might have told you it was a wooden ball painted red, you would end up with a mouth full of splinters.

The feelings you ignore will eventually resurface—unfortunately by that time they are often disguised and displaced by time, harder to recognize, harder to understand, and harder to do something with. The lesson is to listen to your feelings when they appear, and avoid people who are fond of saying "There's no reason to feel that way." Feelings aren't *rational*, there doesn't have to be a logical reason for them. You don't *control* your emotions! What you do control is:

1. What to make of them, how to interpret them, and
2. What to do with them, that is, your own authentic expression or appropriate containment.

Hand in hand with the false notion that feelings should be rational is the common belief that the cure for sadness or despondency is to replace it with pleasant, happy feelings. In fact, the only valid cure for any kind of depression lies in the acceptance of real suffering. To climb out of it any other way is simply a palliative, laying the foundation for the next depression; nothing whatever has happened to the soul.

What I do not advocate is blind positive thinking, but instead a form of "realistic positive thinking." This kind of positive thinking includes crying, sadness, fright, anger, or despair. Allowing the presence of these feelings enhances our ability to feel the good feelings too: joy, laughter, contentment, tranquility, elation, and more. We don't get just the good side without the bad; as a matter of fact, the experience of alternating opposites will enhance our ability to experience life more deeply, with more vitality. And *all* of these states are temporary. When we embrace the inevitability of the bad with the good, this results in "living better," in being the author of your own better quality of life.

In our culture, we may often hear that we should be in control of our lives and of our emotions, that if we are thus in proper control our lives will be good. We are urged to refuse to give in to depressions or fears, instead to keep our chin up and think affirming thoughts. This approach does us a great disservice by denying the ubiquitous, inescapable fact of darkness in our lives. There are times when we indeed should submit to life's suffering, which, when surrendered to, ultimately brings wisdom and authenticity (Sullivan 1989).

By accepting the suffering and demanding no release, we are not excluding a tandem *hope* for release. We hope for a cure, certainly, but more broadly, hope equals living a very full, interesting, productive, worthwhile life with the time you still have, long or short, known or not. Real acceptance plus hope will lead us to seek the appropriate help, whether medication in illness, support of friends in grief, rest in exhaustion, or work either in physical or psychological depression. This attitude is greatly enabled by an awareness that there is always an implicit and universal meaning even in the carrying of small miseries—bearing a tiny part of the darkness of the world (Luke 1995).

Because cancer is a potentially fatal illness and often is characterized by a stigma, cancer patients' network members may withdraw or react inappropriately. Cancer also may affect relationships indirectly by restricting patients' social activities, which will affect their access to interpersonal resources. Many friends and family members have important misconceptions about cancer patients' needs and desires. For example, the majority of support providers tend to say that they would try to cheer up a cancer patient while patients themselves say that others' overdone optimism is quite disturbing. Many caregivers also believe it is harmful for cancer patients to discuss their illness, while patients find it orienting to talk about their cancer, their worries, and their concerns. Also, many healthy people believe that a cancer patient's major concern is cosmetic (losing a breast or having a hysterectomy) but patients' major concerns are more often about cancer recurrence and death, especially at first. Other prominent unhelpful behaviors identified by cancer patients include other people minimizing their difficulties, forced cheerfulness, being told not to worry, medical care being delivered in the absence of emotional support, insensitive comments, and, especially, avoidance of the patient (Helgeson and Cohen 1996). People who behave these ways toward you are best avoided—or, if you're otherwise very fond of them, it may be a worthwhile endeavor to *coach* them in ways you wish them to interact with you.

The perception of receiving good emotional support is strongly associated with hope for the future, a favorable outlook, better emotional adjustment, enhanced role functioning, better self-esteem, higher degree of life satisfaction, and reduced hostility. The different types of supportive interactions, as I touched on before, include emotional, informational, and instrumental support. Emotional support can consist of love, concern, understanding, reassurance, validation, encouragement, listening, physical presence, approval, encouraging expressiveness, empathy, and affection. Instrumental support can consist of aid, assistance, helping with chores, providing transportation, providing child care, medical care, and other practical assistance. Informational support can consist of advice, problem-solving information, telling what to expect, answering questions, and providing a role model. These are things to specifically ask for.

Systems of support do seem to actually prolong life, or at least help substantially with coping . The possible reasons why this is so has to do with the sheer number of important needs that are being addressed by support groups and support networks. These include bolstering a better, more-informed use of health care treatments with encouragement to utilize these well. Another effect is sometimes called the "Grandmother effect"—that is, encouragement to do the things a grandmother might say: eat well, exercise, and sleep well. Group experiences often reduce stress as well: stress secretes hormones that play a role in tumor growth. Likewise, the endocrine or immune system could be enhanced by the group experience. Those in a peer group are the least likely of all support people to minimize talking about the cancer, and they are the most likely to provide validation and understanding. Education is usually part of such a group experience, helping to provide information about cancer effects, treatment options, likely reactions, and giving support for a diversity of responses. This education, according to research studies, seems to provide a particularly strong boost to psychological adjustment—at least as much as, and perhaps even more so than, the emotional support that occurs in support group settings. Educational interventions appear to enhance the patient's perception of control, which in turn is linked to better emotional adjustment. Education may also affect self-esteem and may invite optimism by increasing choices for coping. With this many effects possible, I encourage nearly every woman with cancer to seek out a support group that is to her liking.

When we are living more fully, in tune with our own directions, we will still bump into other peoples' own direction-taking, and things will not always be harmonious. When our travels conflict with another's, it is important to first know what we need for ourselves before we start our socially ingrained compromise and adaptation. This way, the compromise and adaptation will be more authentic: two people negotiating their ways, two people respecting each other's ways and perhaps giving ideas to each other on how best to continue traveling, whether together or divergently.

Remember, *life is hard*. It's *supposed* to be hard. That's just the way of the world. If your life has difficulties, it may not be always because you're doing something wrong. As you keep developing your awareness of your emotional signals and your inner wisdom, the difference between life's given hardships and wise inner signals that something in your life needs your attention becomes more and more clear. This is expressed this way by writer Gillian Rose as she struggles with the meaning of her ovarian cancer:

> Exceptional, edgeless love effaces the risk of rela-
> tion: that mix of exposure and reserve, of reve-
> lation and reticence. It commands the complete
> unveiling of the eyes, the transparency of the body.
> . . . Existence is robbed of its weight, its gravity,
> when it is deprived of its agon. Instead of insinu-
> ating that illness may better prepare you for the
> earthly impossibilities. These enchiridions of
> Faith, Hope, and Love would condemn you to seek
> blissful, deathless, cosmic emptiness — the repose
> without the revel.
>
> I reach for my favorite whisky bottle and in-
> struct my valetudinarian well-wishers to imbibe
> the shark's oil and aloe vera themselves. If I am to
> stay alive, I am bound to continue to get love
> wrong, all the time, but not to cease wooing, for
> that is my life affair, my *love's work*. [Rose 1995]

ENVISIONING THE SELF

A woman's cancer can often be the turning point for a woman to reenvision her life. She is likely to reenvision her purpose, her values, and her identity. These existential acts usually encompass new definitions of masculinity and femininity. Particularly, women with cancer can often see a broader picture of self, one that no longer views masculinity and femininity as mutually exclusive, nor even as opposites. Rather, masculinity and femininity are seen as simply traits that call out various forms of experience and expression, some of which are to be cultivated, some of which are to be let alone to recede. These choices no longer need to be driven by gender stereotypes. The modern preference for understanding and control, for information and manipulation are considered traditional masculine values. Instead, or, better yet, in addition to this practical way of living, women can add feminine approaches for living, for nourishing the soul: living from senses of imagination, enchantment, entrancement, rapture, being spirited away and spellbound, being caring and receptive and intuitive. A whole person is one who can incorporate traits from several sources instead of just one. Doing so gives us much more access to all our potentialities.

A woman's cancer, its treatments, and its aftermath call for a woman to become more of what is typically considered masculine: to explore her surroundings and ask for information, to actively advocate for herself, to aggressively fight (a disease in this case), and to reduce the typically female traits of focusing on appearance for acceptance and for being pretty, soft, receptive, sweet, and pleasing. This reevaluation and rebalancing allows a woman to decide for herself which traditionally feminine and which traditionally masculine traits she will value and embody.

At this time in her life, a woman can turn from the often hidden contempt for the traditional feminine values so that she may cease to identify her worth, her creativity, solely with the traditional masculine productions of thought and with achievements in the outer world. For example, a woman who quietly *responds* with intense interest and love to people, to ideas, and to things is as deeply and truly creative and alive as one who always seeks to lead, to act, to achieve. The feminine qualities of responsiveness and receptivity and of nurturing in silence are (whether in man or woman) as essential to creation as their masculine counterparts and in no way inferior (Luke 1995). We are now free to redevelop our receptive side.

> If we can rediscover in ourselves the hidden beauty of this *receptive devotion* (italics mine), if we can learn how to be still without inaction, how to 'further life' without willed purpose, how to serve without demanding prestige, and how to nourish without domination: then we shall be women again out of whose earth the light may shine. [Luke 1995]

What becomes essential is the ability of a woman to validate her own convictions of truth, beauty, and goodness in regard to her self-concept and self-interest. Body image, self-confidence, personal agency, social functioning, occupational functioning, sexual pleasure, and subjective self-assessment are all related to this ability. The experience of being one's own agent, that is, the owner of one's own will, is a key factor in securing a personal identity and is a major concern for women growing into psychological health. An adult's recognition of competence, perceived control, or personal agency is the unifying element in being a person-among-persons, a viable individual and member of society.

Fundamental to having a coherent identity is the knowledge that one does things effectively, that one is useful. To act with intention, with responsibility, with free choice is personal agency. Also, economic independence and work competence are core factors of personal agency, personal efficacy. Having work that is challenging and imaginative, and having a personal sovereignty over one's finances, are also basic to maintaining the experience of perceived control. The post-cancer woman may find herself re-creating these. And, rather than maintaining a consistent set of self-attributes which she imposes on all situations, a woman can strive for an ability to be both empathic and decisive in her responses to each new environment while she maintains a commitment to her own values (Young-Eisendrath and Wiedemann 1987).

Because she has faced incredible uncertainties, a woman with a woman's cancer comes to a better position for finding a way to achieve a symbolic immortality, something we may all need to do. Women accomplish this in many ways. Acquiring symbolic immortality may happen via:

1. The Biologic Mode—living through one's descendants;
2. The Theological Mode—living on in a different, higher plane of existence;
3. The Creative Mode—living on through one's works, one's personal creations, or one's impact on others;
4. The theme of Eternal Nature—one survives through rejoining the swirling life forces of nature;

5. The Experiential Transcendent Mode—through "losing oneself" in a state so intense that time and death disappear and one lives in the "continuous present" (Yalom 1980).

My women patients, and their loved ones, have described an amazing collection of manifestations of a higher being or higher sense that guides their way. Some of these are the following: the Catholic or Christian Holy Virgin (who intercedes at the time of death to help one step across the gulf), the African Goddess Oya (a protector who can manifest in motion, activity, wind), the Egyptian Goddess Isis (known as The Great Mother and Healer), the Hindu Shakti (the creative primal feminine principle that energizes all divinity, every being, and every thing), Nature and Shaman Healers, Hindu Kali (the Virgin-Creator, Sustaining Mother, and Absorber-Destroyer), Chinese Kuan Yin (Goddess of Mercy), Tibetan Buddhist Dakini (the energizing feminine principle), God, Yaweh, and Allah, among others. Also, many women mention the importance of their spiritual practices: Christian Science healing, Quaker Stillness, Taoism, meditation, imagery, rituals, saying the rosary, homage to ancestors, (political) activism, a macrobiotic diet, Jewish Kashrut, fasting, Zen Shojin, growing your own food, Sufism, Native American sweat lodge or smudging. These many forms of a higher sense or helping entity are wonderful companions to many women on a cancer journey, both as healing guides and as possible paths to symbolic immortality.

Some people believe that diseases of the body are often attributable to an imbalance in life. The imbalance

sometimes originates within the body or spirit and sometimes in the outside world. Either way, what is central to
healing is *relationship with the rest of creation.* Cure begins and
ends with relationship. The purpose of ceremony is to
restore the individual to her place within all the rest, recon-
necting and restoring the human body with earth, with
cosmos. To have health, it is necessary to keep all these re-
lations in mind, to create a relationship with other people,
with animals, with the land. The body, made of earth's mud
and breathed into with life, is considered the temple, and
we can learn to worship it as such, to move slowly within it,
listening, respecting it, loving it, treating ourselves and all
our loved ones with tenderness. And the love for the body
and for the earth are, to many people, the same love (Hogan
1994).

To re-create your place within the world becomes a primal force post cancer. We do so as women, and we do so
within our parameters of health—physical, mental, emotional, and spiritual. To re-create our femininity and womanliness we ask ourselves to make explicit our prior definitions: did femininity mean being overly nice? We may change
this to being simply *very* nice, and nice to ourselves as much
as to others. Did womanhood mean too much work and not
enough play? We may rebalance these quantitatively. Did
femininity and womanhood connote fraility, emotionality,
overconcern with appearance, vulnerability, trying to elicit
rather than solicit what you want from others? We may
recalibrate the degree of our expression of each of these
traits. Did your former definitions of femininity and womanhood contain qualities you clearly want to continue to

own, such as strength or ability to serve others or intuitive perceptions? We may certainly keep these, and continue to enhance them. We don't have to make a complete 180 degree turn around of our prior definitions. Our changes may instead be simple, well thought out modifications.

In this same vein, we may take inventory of the coping devices and emotional signals we used prior to cancer in order to make a reevaluation. Did you formerly surprise yourself with undue irritability sometimes? You may now read that as a meaningful signal from your psyche to change the sources of irritation, change your approach to them, or add soothing and replenishing activities to counter the irritants. Were your former primary coping devices denial, overcompensation, displacement, and unremitting worry? You may want too keep some of these available in your tool box, but use them less often as you increase your use of coping devices that may serve you better in the long run, such as mastery, substitution, searching for meaningfulness, and cultivating social networks. Was the former you less able to grieve, less able to express yourself, more the reader rather than the author of your life's story? Your post-cancer reevaluation cannot help but give you more ability to have an impact on your own quality of life.

A reevaluation of the personal meaning of the organs, body parts, physical appearance, and physical abilities that are the outcome of your cancer can also take you to new, more psychologically healthy places. You may take a loving, deeply earnest inventory of the meaning, use, and impact of these body capacities and their changes. Your breasts, your reproductive organs, your genitalia, or any affected diges-

tive organs may have special and important symbolic significance to you as a human and especially as a woman. Finding these meanings allows an awesome unfolding to occur.
You may then grieve the losses and changes fully, because
you have thoroughly named the meaning of the losses. You
are then more able to invent renewed ways to reestablish
similar meaningfulness in your life. This process, this task,
becomes for many women the very foundation upon which
they can rebuild a satisfying sense of self and place in the
world; this is usually a place of substantially more empow-
erment, efficacy, and contentment than we ever knew was
possible prior to cancer.

Nearly everything a woman needs to live her life to her
highest potential already resides within her. The task,
whether accomplished via a therapist, spiritual guide, friend,
spouse, or on her own, is to mobilize and actualize her own
health rather than to cure her. This is a process already trying to happen. Within herself, or with the help of others, a
woman can coax out a developmental line, feed and water
the seeds of her growth that lie dormant in the depths of
her soul, and smooth the path for her growth into light. After
having a woman's cancer, and while navigating the recovery
process, whether emotional or physical, a woman comes to
more completely own, operate, and manage her life. The
price of this ownership is that daily she faces new choices
that require a vigilant responsibility for the ongoing expression of her own vision. These existential acts form the soil
of the soul, where she can evermore plant her chosen seeds,
balance her needs with those of others, struggle with the

ever-present weeds, and come to some terms with the meaning of her garden, of her life.

Choice is difficult. This is so because it requires facing any "wasted" prior time. Because it means committing to a course of action. Because it means relinquishing one possibility at a time as one chooses another. Because it means we are accountable and cannot put blame elsewhere.

> Fear is a poor excuse for not doing the work. We are all afraid. It is nothing new. If you are alive, you are fearful. [Estés 1992]

Fear is an inherent part of facing life full on. Courage does not mean having no fear. Courage means feeling the fear and finding a way through it. Healing comes not from a removal of the conflicts that were the cause of existential pain but precisely from realizing the reality of the conflicts—and by a full and free acceptance of the suffering this brings. We all face the same essential problems throughout our lives: what we call problems of intimacy, of closeness and distance from others, of the need to be our own separate selves at the same time as we attach to and unite with other human beings. Each person works out the insoluble strains and paradoxes in her own way, and continually over her lifetime.

We have a gift beyond measure, the daily bliss of being alive. Forced by our disease to "walk through the valley of the shadow of death," like any woman who gives birth, we get to experience the sacredness of life—and the thin line between life and death. Cancer is real life, our real life. When you know you walk this earth on borrowed time, each day can be a beloved friend. You notice the small beauties, the cycles and seasons, you celebrate color and season and texture; you see the dark sides and the trivial and float through them as part of the riches of a balanced life.

Finding a truer, stronger voice is the antidote to despair, to fear of death, to constricted living. Speaking more clearly than perhaps we did before cancer, that is what helps us live life more meaningfully, more zestfully. We can throw off the old constricture, "Nice girls don't . . . " as in, nice girls don't "talk about that," don't "act like that," don't "have desires or needs." Thus, we can also check our reality, or experiences, against those of others. This can bring relief, or aid, or a renewed inner balance.

> Frankly, I don't expect that vitamin C or shark liver oil or seaweed by itself will save my life, any more than chemotherapy alone will. In my heart I feel that what *will* save my life is the journey to a richer, deeper connection to life. [Hooper 1994]

Being human is really about having fire, flair, a holy spark of inspiration. For a woman with a woman's cancer, her ideal becomes the development of an equilibrium between effort and pleasure, between mind and passion, between receptivity and power. A sense of belonging and natural inheritance is what we long for—the comfort that comes from being cradled by a continuity, the freedom from insignificance. How much time and energy we must spend just claiming an ordinary place for ourselves! We must re-

invent ourselves every day. How to choose from all the identity options available to us! Sometimes we are faint from ex-
cess, paralyzed by choice. The claustrophobia of no choice
versus the agoraphobia of open options—it is difficult to dis-
entangle fashionable views from true belief, passionate con-
viction from defensive dogma (Hoffman 1989). Yet these
are the tasks of maturation. We try our best to age into these
tasks gracefully, to "Sing oneself through a hard experience,
not sing oneself *out* of it," as opera singer Jessye Norman
describes it. With aging comes the call to embrace adversity
with elegance.

> Many women hovering near fifty have whispered
> to me and I to them of how the world opens up,
> of the mysterious change, the surge of freedom,
> the possibility of new adventures, indeed of birth,
> when they can say, "I am not young, I do not want
> to be young, I do not want men to look at me as
> though I were young. My life no longer starts with
> my body, with how I look. In the spectrum of
> camouflage, I am now at the far end with no cam-
> ouflage whatever. I have gray hair that I keep in a
> bun and I wear glasses, but who I am is what I do,
> what I say, and whom I love. I have passed through
> the magic circle of invisibility into a new life."
> [Heilbrun 1996]

Both by our aging and our standing up to our cancer
we are reminded that we do not wish our worth to be judged
primarily by our appearance, as may have occurred in our

former definition of our femininity. Rather, we come to value our inner strengths, our health, our ability to act effectively, our endurance, our highly adequate skills at navigating life's rough roads as well as the smooth ones. These seal our worth.

When we travel deeply enough, we encounter an elemental sadness, for full awareness of ourselves always includes the knowledge of our own ephemerality and the passage of time. But it is only in that knowledge—not its denial—that experiences gain their true dimensions, and we can feel the simplicity of being alive. It is only that knowledge that is large enough to cradle a tenderness for everything that is always to be lost—a tenderness for each of our moments, for others, and for the world. The ontological guilt, as the existentialists call it—not fulfilling our potentials—does not so much lead to paralysis or symptoms; instead it can lead to humility, to sensitivity in one's relationships, and increased creativity in the use of one's potentialities (May 1983).

๑๑

Cancer.

It will now be an integral part of each of us forevermore.

It will have thrown us to the ground, and been a source of our recovery into ways of living that we may resonate to much, much better.

Our cancer may leave bodily scars, but we will refocus our body image in ways that shine our inner light visibly onto others and into the darkness.

Our cancer may seem to rob us of our femininity, our womanliness, only to become the soil from which sprouts an embracing of our cherished feminine qualities—perhaps intuition, emotionality, or beauty—and a cultivation of masculine traits we once thought we shouldn't have—such as being direct or actively standing up for ourselves.

Our cancer may compromise our physical fertility, yet becomes a bridge to an *internalized* sense of fertility, purpose, womanliness, and attractiveness.

Our cancer forces us to question the quality of our caring and the ways others care for us, resulting in a renewed balance where love and care of ourselves is given in equal proportion to love and care of others.

Our cancer takes us through one of the biggest fears we've ever known, yet teaches us how to greet our fear as a constant companion, thus lessening its power to shake us up.

Our cancer tears us apart from our bodies, challenges our spirituality, and questions our mind's view of our lives, then reunites our parts into a more authentic embodied–mindful–spirited woman.

Our cancer saps our vitality and removes us from ourselves as we listen to a hundred opinions about what we should do, then fills us with the energy to remake a new vitality within new confines and to listen to our own voice for guidance.

Our cancer puts blinders on our eyes, narrowing our vision to cope with the emergency, then removes the blinders and asks us to expand our vision further than ever before to accept the task of making our own meaning out of life's shifting sands.

Our cancer transforms itself from something we hate into a reason to cherish ourselves, and by cherishing ourselves, we find that we are valuable, and can begin to act in ways that express our values.

Thank you, cancer.

> In the bowels of the hospital, or the receding world that illness creates, or in the fearful half-light of the psychological underworld, patients . . . reach the point of realizing that their old self and old life are dead, at least for now, perhaps forever. For the soul, this can be a turning point: facing the possibility of disability or death can be reorienting, it can bring about a massive change in priorities, and bring to the forefront questions of meaning and meaninglessness about how we are living our lives, about what really matters, and whether we matter. For the ego that had maintained the illusion of control over fate, this is often the lowest point. For the person, if ego turns to soul to lead the way through the underworld, there will be unexpected discoveries. For *it's not what happens to us, but how we respond that ultimately matters* and shapes who we are from inside out. [Bolen 1996]

∞

We are all dying. The dying have a responsibility to the living: to leave a legacy. Whether we are to die soon or far from now, we must search out the sources of our cancers and fight for our lives and the lives of young women rising up after us. We must be an active tool in this fight, not waiting for others to do it for us. There are many paths open to us to accomplish this. The choices are yours to make.

You may want to start with a deeper finding of yourself by taking an inventory: Do you like to sleep with the windows open or closed? Do you prefer wilderness or cities? Do you move fast or slowly? Do you prefer details or the big picture? Which of your senses is most adept at drinking in the world? Do you want a life partner? Children? Great grandchildren? Community? Are you more adventuresome or timid? What are your least favorite ways of behaving? Which talents and skills do you want to cultivate? Which plants, music, arts, literature, sports, terrains, modes of travel, foods, animals mean the most to you? What does your womanhood mean to you, your femininity? What do you think is your reason for being in this life? What legacy would you like to leave behind? How shall you nourish your own vision?

From a place of knowing yourself this well – and you will ask these questions again and again over your lifetime to stay in touch with yourself—you will create methods for living your life in the best ways for you. And that cancer of yours—it will tug at you to *do* something about it once you've realized how much you've learned from it. What can you do with it? From the very personal methods to the very political, why not start with enrolling in a clinical trial?

What is a clinical trial? Randomized clinical trials are studies that are designed to compare the outcome of two or more different treatments. Besides randomized trials, which are designed to randomly assign participants to different treatment modes, other types of research design are being conducted. For example, case-control studies are ones in which a group of people with cancer is compared with a group of people who do not have cancer; the studies look for differences in health behavior, medication history, biochemical measures, and other measures. Another type of study design, called cohort design, are long range studies in which information is collected on a group who have been exposed to a suspected substance or behavior, and these people are followed for many years to see who gets cancer and who does not.

Clinical trials for cancer can be sponsored by the National Cancer Institute, an academic institution, or private industry. In these studies, usually a newer, promising treatment is compared with a well-established treatment so that the outcomes can be compared. This also assures that no matter which of the two treatments a participant is assigned to, she will be receiving good treatment. Usually the cost of the treatment is free to you. Often these studies are "double-blind," which means that neither the doctors nor the patients know which treatment the patients are actually receiving. This will be revealed at the end of the study. The double-blind method eliminates bias from the study; it also points out how powerfully our minds can affect treatment outcomes when we already know what treatment we are receiving (this phenomenon has been shown repeatedly in studies). There is no better way known to test the benefits of new treatments. It can be very difficult to not know what you are being treated with, yet enrolling in a clinical trial not only provides you with one of the better treatments known, but it will benefit cancer survivors who come after you. Call the National Cancer Institute (1-800-4-CANCER) or the Woman's Health Initiative (1-800-54-WOMEN) or ask your doctor about enrolling in a clinical trial.

We can't really criticize the lack of needed research and information on women's cancers unless we do something about it individually. In addition to clinical trials and other studies, there are innumerable ways for each woman to make her mark on the cancer world:

- Donate money to cancer organizations.
- Actively raise money for cancer organizations.
- Get into political action on cancer.
- Become a mentor to other cancer survivors.
- Write about cancer to newspapers, legislators, friends, or the company newsletter.
- Promote art about cancer.
- Give talks about cancer.
- Volunteer at a hospital or cancer center.
- Share the effects of your cancer on your spiritual life.
- Be a courageous model for those who will come after you.
- Promote cancer screening and information to minority women and poor women.
- Keep up the pressure.
- Leave an imprint.

Resources

National Cancer Institute
    Fact sheets from NCI, current clinical information, publications, news. Supports many cancer centers throughout the country.
        Phone: 1-800-4-CANCER
        Internet gopher site: CancerNet
American Cancer Society
    Pamphlets, information sheets, help with breast prostheses, workplace and insurance information. Has divisions in every state.
        Phone: 1-800-ACS-2345
Canadian Cancer Information Service
    Information and answers to treatment questions, research, and statistics.
        Phone: 1-800-263-6750

National Alliance of Breast Cancer Organizations
   Excellent list of resources, fact sheets, quarterly newsletter, events, local support groups, and referrals to sources of information about clinical trials.
      Phone: 1-212-719-0154
Susan G. Komen Foundation
   National help-line for breast cancer resources. Sponsors the Race for the Cure.
      Phone: 1-800-I'M-AWARE
Women's Health Initiative
   A major research study of women and their health, examining how diet, hormone therapy, and calcium and vitamin D might prevent heart disease, breast and colorectal cancers, and bone fractures in women over 50 years of age.
      Sponsored by the National Institutes of Health
      Phone: 1-800-54-WOMEN

References

Atkinson, D. A. (1994). Breast Cancer and the Adjustment Process. Dissertation.

Austin, S., and Hitchcock, K. (1994). *Breast Cancer: What You Should Know (But May Not Be Told) About Prevention, Diagnosis, and Treatment.* Rocklin, CA: Prima Publications.

Bateson, M. C. (1989). *Composing a Life.* New York: Penguin.

Bepko, C., and Krestan, J. (1993). *Singing at the Top of Our Lungs.* New York: Harper Perennial.

Bolen, J. S. (1996). *Close to the Bone: Life-Threatening Illness and the Search for Meaning.* New York: Scribner.

Bowen, D. (1994). *Cancer and Cancer Risk Among Lesbians.* Proceedings of An Interactive Working Conference, Fred Hutchinson Cancer Research Center, Seattle, WA, December.

Compas, B. E., Worsham, N. L., Ey, S., and Howell, D. C. (1996). When mom or dad has cancer II: coping, cognitive appraisals, and psychological distress in children of cancer patients. *Health Psychology* 15(3):167–175.

Coping. (1995). The BRCA1 breast cancer susceptibility gene. p. 54.

Estés, C. P. (1992). *Women Who Run with the Wolves.* New York: Ballantine.

Greenspan, M. (1983). *A New Approach to Women and Therapy.* New York: McGraw-Hill.

Harvard women's health watch. (1996). *Women's Health Studies.* September, p. 6.

Helgeson, V. S. and Cohen, S. (1996). Social support and adjustment to cancer: reconciling descriptive, correlational, and intervention research. *Health Psychology.* 15(2):135–148.

Heilbrun, C. (1996). Coming of age. In *The Seasons of Women,* ed. G. Norris, pp. 428–431. New York: Norton.

Herman, J. L. (1992). *Trauma and Recovery.* New York: Basic Books.

Hoffman, E. (1989). *Lost in Translation.* New York: Penguin.

Hogan, L. (1994). Department of the interior. In *Minding the Body,* ed. P. Foster, pp. 159–174. New York: Anchor.

Holland, J. C., and Rowland, J. H. (eds.). (1989). *Handbook of Psychooncology: Psychological Care of the Patient with Cancer.* New York: Oxford University Press. 1991.

Holling, S. (1996). Letters. *Ms. Magazine.* VII(1): pp. 4–5.

Hooper, J. (1994). Beauty tips for the dead. In *Minding the Body,* ed. P. Foster, pp. 107–137. New York: Anchor.

Jordan, J. V., and Surrey, J. L. (1986). The self in relation: empathy and the mother daughter relationship. In *The Psychology of Today's Woman*, ed. T. Bernay and D. W. Cantor, pp. 81–104. Hillsdale, N. J.: Analytic Press.

Kaschak, E. (1992). *Engendered Lives.* New York: Basic Books.

Kaye, R. (1991). *Spinning Straw Into Gold.* New York: Simon & Schuster.

King, M. C. (1996). Komen-funded research leads to important discovery in genetics of breast cancer. *Front Line Newsletter.* Susan G. Komen Breast Cancer Foundation. Spring.

Kolodzie, M. E. (1996). Women's sexual functioning during and after menopause: an overview. *The Health Psychologist.* 18(3): 4–19.

Krakoff, I. H. (1996). Systemic treatment of cancer. *CA.* 46(3): 134–141.

Lasry, J. M. and Margolese, R. G. (1991). Fear of recurrence, breast conserving surgery, and the trade-off hypothesis. *CA.* 69(8): pp. 2111–2115.

Lerner, H. G. (1988). *Women and Therapy.* New York: Harper & Row.

Lorde, A. (1980). *The Cancer Journals.* San Francisco: Spinsters/ Aunt Lute.

Louden, J. (1992). *The Woman's Comfort Book.* New York: HarperCollins.

Love, S. (1991). *Dr. Susan Love's Breast Book.* Reading, MA: Addison-Wesley.

Luke, H. M. (1995). *The Way of Woman.* New York: Doubleday.

Maddi, S. (1990). Prolonging life by heroic measures. In *Psychological Aspects of Serious Illness*, ed. P. Costa and G. VandenBos. Washington, DC: American Psychological Association.

May, R. (1983). *The Discovery of Being.* New York: Norton.

Miller, S. M., Rodoletz, M., Schroeder, C. M., Mangan, C. E., and Sedlacek, T.V. (1996). Applications of the monitoring process model to coping with severe long-term medical threats. *Health Psychology.* 15(3):216–225.

Mitchell, S. A. (1993). *Hope and Dread in Psychoanalysis.* New York: Basic Books.

Nesse, R. M., and Williams, G. C. (1994) . *Why We Get Sick.* New York: Times.

Oxenhandler, N. (1995). Fruits of the Body. *Vogue.* June, pp. 56–62.

Parker, S. L., Tong, T., Bolden, S., & Wingo, P. A. (1996). Cancer Statistics, 1996. *CA.* 46(1): pp. 5–27.

————. (1997). Cancer Statistics, 1997. *CA.* 47(1): pp. 5–27.

Rose, G. (1995). *Love's Work.* New York: Schocken Books.

Rosser, S. V. (1994). *Women's Health—Missing from U. S. Medicine.* Bloomington: Indiana University Press.

Runowicz, C. D., and Haupt, D. (1995). *To Be Alive.* New York: Henry Holt.

Schover, L. R. (1991). The impact of breast cancer on sexuality, body image, and intimate relationships. *CA.* 41(2) pp. 112–120.

Small, E. C. (1994). Psychosocial-sexual issues. *Obstetrics and Gynecology Clinics of North America* 21:773–780.

Sullivan, B. S. (1989). *Psychotherapy Grounded in the Feminine Principle.* Wilmette, IL: Chiron.

Taylor, S. (1990). Psychological aspects of chronic illness. In *Psychological Aspects of Serious Illness*, ed. P. Costa and G. VandenBos. Washington, DC: American Psychological Association.

Travis, C. B. (1988). *Women and Health Psychology: Biomedical Issues.* New York: Lawrence Erlbaum.

Weisman, A. D., and Worden, J. W. (1976–1977). The existential plight in cancer: significance of the first 100 days. *International Journal of Psychiatry in Medicine* 7:1–15.

Williams, T. T. (1991). *Refuge.* New York: Pantheon.

Yalom, I. D. (1980). *Existential Psychotherapy.* New York: Basic Books.

Young-Eisendrath, P., and Wiedemann, F. L. (1987). *Female Authority.* New York: Guilford.

Index